Water Exercise

Martha D. White, OTR
Therapeutic Alternatives
Houston, Texas

Human Kinetics

To my Mom and Dad and my mentor, the late Roy Don Wilson, ATC

Library of Congress Cataloging-in-Publication Data

White, Martha, 1956-
    Water exercise / Martha White.
        p.   cm.
    Includes index.
    ISBN: 0-87322-726-3
    1. Water exercises.   I. Title.
    RA781.17.W45   1995
    615.8'53--dc20

75523

94-44193
CIP

ISBN: 0-87322-726-3

Developmental Editors: Mary E. Fowler and Dawn Roselund; **Assistant Editor:** Henry Woolsey; **Copyeditor:** Rita Doyle; **Proofreader:** Lee Erwin; **Indexer:** Sheila Ary; **Typesetting and Layout:** Ruby Zimmerman; **Text Design:** Judy Henderson; **Cover Design:** Keith Blomberg; **Photographer (cover):** Nate Fine; **Illustrator:** Dianna Porter; **Printer:** United Graphics

Human Kinetics books are available at special discounts for bulk purchase. Special editions or book excerpts can also be created to specification. For details, contact the Special Sales Manager at Human Kinetics.

Printed in the United States of America   10   9   8   7   6   5   4   3   2   1

Human Kinetics
P.O. Box 5076, Champaign, IL 61825-5076
1-800-747-4457

Canada: Human Kinetics, Box 24040, Windsor, ON N8Y 4Y9
1-800-465-7301 (in Canada only)

Europe: Human Kinetics, P.O. Box IW14, Leeds LS16 6TR, England
(44) 532 781708

Australia: Human Kinetics, 2 Ingrid Street, Clapham 5062, South Australia
(08) 371 3755

New Zealand: Human Kinetics, P.O. Box 105-231, Auckland 1
(09) 309 2259

Contents

foreword

The most important ingredient for successful recovery from any musculoskeletal condition is rehabilitation, which often requires strenuous and painful exercise regimens in order for the patient to regain strength and motion in the affected part. Progress may be slow, and the patient may give up on his or her therapy if too much pain is involved.

Water therapy is an excellent method to use when normal gravity conditions might make the rehabilitation process difficult, painful, and even dangerous. For several years Martha White has shown me the value of water therapy in my patients, and I am glad that she is now sharing her experience in this book. Using any of the exercise protocols described here will greatly help the injured patient in his or her recovery.

In this book, Martha also has included descriptions of water exercises for the healthy person. Benefits of working out in a water environment include strengthening, development of muscle symmetry, cross-training, weight reduction, reduction of blood pressure and cholesterol levels, and improved overall health. Most of us early in life are able to accomplish these goals in normal training and under normal gravity conditions. However, as we get older, we develop afflictions in our musculoskeletal systems. By using a water exercise program we can maintain a fitness level without being too hard on our bodies.

I congratulate Martha on her excellent presentation in this book.

Leland Winston, MD
Orthopaedic Surgeon
Houston, Texas

Preface

Welcome to the world of water exercise! Congratulations for your consideration of water as an avenue for rehabilitation or preventive fitness. In the following pages, many questions concerning specific water exercise programs for injuries, postsurgical rehabilitation, fitness, or crosstraining are answered. Each area is addressed from the beginning to advanced phases to ensure better results and prevent possible injury or aggravation of symptoms. You will be guided through each exercise with a concise, descriptive text and an accompanying illustration.

This book is for everyone, including the individual recuperating from surgery to the back or an extremity, the sedentary person starting an exercise program who needs a guiding hand, the athlete desiring a crosstraining program to enhance athletic performance, or the individual who wants to lose some weight and gain muscle tone. Anyone can benefit from the exercise programs presented in the following pages. Whether you are a beginner in water exercise or a competitive athlete, an appropriate program for your needs is included within this book.

In Part I, the benefits of water exercise for therapy or fitness are discussed. The properties of water that make it a good therapeutic environment are discussed, as well as the overall physical rehabilitative benefits of exercise in the water. Steps necessary for water exercise are also covered. The various pieces of equipment used throughout the text are highlighted, with information on manufacturing or retail sources included as well.

In Part II, you will be introduced to a myriad of exercises from beginning, intermediate, and advanced levels, with detailed text to talk you through each exercise. Illustrations accompany the text to ensure reader comprehension and safety at all times. These exercises are detailed in chapters 3, 4, and 5. Chapter 6 discusses and illustrates deep water exercises from beginner to advanced levels.

Water is an excellent medium for rehabilitation from any type of injury or surgery. Injury-specific programs are addressed in chapters 7, 8, 9, 10, 11, and 12 of Part III and cover the major joints of the body, as well as the trunk and spine. Each chapter in Part III addresses injuries or surgeries common to a specific joint and outlines an exercise program from beginner to advanced levels to be followed in the water.

Part IV of *Water Exercise* covers water exercise for total fitness from a beginner level to an advanced cross-training program. The final chapter of the book is devoted to special populations, including people with rheumatoid arthritis, osteoporosis, Parkinsonism, and fibromyalgia. A fitness program is presented for those with special needs.

There are great possibilities with water exercise when it is followed on a consistent, structured basis. Proceed at a safe and comfortable pace. You did not get where you are overnight, so you cannot expect spectacular changes overnight. Be smart with your body.

I wish you the very best with your water exercise program for therapy or fitness. I commend you for taking an active role in your health and recovery. Good luck, and enjoy yourself in your new fitness and health endeavor.

Acknowledgments

First, I would like to thank all those patients I have worked with in my pool program for their support and encouragement. They are a continuous source of inspiration to me. Also, a big thanks to Randy James of J-Art for the great job on the original illustrations. Thanks to Mark Brandt for preparing the text; your humor and attention to detail saved me. Thanks also to the editorial staff of Human Kinetics, especially Mary Fowler. I really appreciate my family for their patience and continuous encouragement along the way. Thanks also to those therapists, nurses, and doctors who recognize water therapy for its many healing qualities and were open to trying it as a therapeutic alternative for their patients. I appreciate the input and support of my co-workers and the physicians associated with Hermann Hospital Sports Medicine Clinic and the greater Houston area. Most of all, I thank God for the opportunity to teach and instruct others in this form of rehabilitation and enable them to improve their quality of life and move forward to a better place. This book is dedicated to all those individuals whose lives have been and will be enriched through water therapy.

Part I

Water Exercise, Therapy, and Fitness

At some point, you may have heard that water is great for rehabilitation or overall fitness, but no one ever told you why or how. In chapter 1 you'll discover the many reasons why water speeds the healing process and enhances overall health. You'll learn about how the properties of water make workouts easier and less painful to do than land exercises, making water an excellent avenue for therapy and fitness.

Specific exercises and program designs are discussed in chapter 2, along with an introduction to various pieces of water exercise equipment now available commercially. Information on where equipment can be obtained also is included.

Now that you are seriously considering water exercise for therapeutic or fitness reasons, come with me and take the plunge into the exciting and increasingly popular world of water exercise.

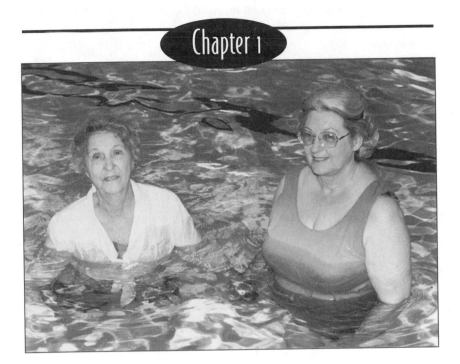

Chapter 1

The Many Benefits of Water Exercise

Water is an excellent medium for therapy for recovery from minor to major injuries, surgery, and for cross-training or preventive fitness. It decreases the wear and tear on the body from leisure or competitive sports or job-related duties. It addresses muscle imbalances or postural problems that may lead to recurrent, nagging injuries from the over-development of muscle groups that are used repetitively.

Nagging injuries can develop from work patterns and recreational sports. If unaddressed, they can evolve into a chronic pattern or a major disruptive injury.

The ever-increasing symptoms need to be tended to in a timely manner to avoid a disruptive development or injury in the future. In this instance, water exercise is so effective because it offers such a wide range of therapeutic and health care benefits, especially when compared with other physical activities. Before you undertake a water exercise program, examine the following list. If you have any of these conditions, you might be prevented from participation, or you will at least need medical clearance before entering the water:

- Open wounds
- Infectious skin conditions
- Severe hypertension or hypotension
- Chemical allergies to pool products
- Seizures
- Diminished respiratory capacity
- Surgical sutures
- Bladder or vaginal infections

THE PROPERTIES OF WATER

Any one of the several characteristics of water alone is therapeutic, and the combination of these properties makes water more comprehensive and beneficial than land exercises for rehabilitation and fitness. Let us examine these properties individually to better understand their effects on us physically.

- **Buoyancy.** Buoyancy is the upward pressure exerted by the fluid in which the body is immersed. Buoyancy opposes the force of gravity, allowing the body to move more freely and easily than on land.

- **Decreased Compressive Forces.** Again, this is due to the effects of buoyancy. The deeper one is in water, the greater the decrease in the compressive or weight-bearing forces on all joints, as well as the discs of the spine.

- **Even Hydrostatic Pressure on Submerged Body Parts.** There is equal pressure from the water on the body that increases with depth. This is helpful for swelling around the joints or circulatory problems because the static fluid around the joints is forced upward toward the heart by hydrostatic pressure.

EXERCISING FOR REHABILITATION

The properties of water are ideal for achieving therapeutic goals in a safe and effective environment. Many individuals who are unable to do their rehabilitation in a conventional clinic setting can successfully participate in a water exercise program. Restrictions from recent surgery or chronic pain are better accommodated in water because of the supportive and gravity-reduced environment.

• **Flexibility.** Due to the decrease of gravitational forces in the water, the body moves freely and the overall weight is diminished so that a body part, such as a leg, can be lifted and stretched without as much pain. Good flexibility is a primary component in recovery from injury or surgery.

• **Muscle Re-education.** When the mechanics of movement of the body, specifically the arm or leg, have been altered through injury or surgery, that area must be taught to move again in accordance with the rest of the body. Another example of impaired movement patterns is limbs that have been immobilized through casting or bracing, or by a stroke. The weakened area is supported through buoyancy and thus more easily and less painfully rehabilitated.

• **Increase in Range of Motion.** Again, the body part or extremity that has experienced loss of full motion can be rehabilitated in water's supportive, gravity-reduced environment. These properties allow the individual to push that joint further toward its goal of full motion with less pain overall.

• **Strengthening.** The arm or leg that has been casted or braced will gain strength in the water because in whatever direction it is moved, it will be working against resistance. This is true for the back surgery patient, stroke patient, or multiple sclerosis patient, among others.

• **Balance Control.** Overall balance is enhanced by moving forward, backward, and sideways in a dynamic (or constantly moving) environment. Not only is the environment ever-changing, but the individual is also always moving in this multidirectional, resistive environment.

• **Safety.** The primary attraction of water as a therapeutic environment is overall safety. Water is supportive through buoyancy, resistive in nature, and equal in hydrostatic pressure on the submerged body part. Weakness, joint or limb swelling, loss of motion or flexibility, and overall loss of endurance are safely addressed in the aquatic environment.

• **Decrease in Spasticity.** Individuals dealing with any degree of spasticity as a result of strokes, cerebral palsy, Parkinson's disease, or multiple sclerosis, to name a few, will have a reduction in muscle tone. They will be able to move more freely in the water. The raising of the body's temperature and warming of the muscles through circulatory responses result in the decrease of spasticity in warmer water.

EXERCISING FOR FITNESS

Water exercise is multifaceted. Not only is it a comprehensive therapeutic tool, it has far-reaching positive health benefits as well. Some of the same advantages of water exercise for rehabilitation are also available when exercising for fitness. These include gains in strength, range of motion, and flexibility. There are other reasons to choose water exercise to improve the overall level of fitness.

• **Muscle Symmetry.** To prevent injuries in competitive or leisure sports, comparable strength in all muscle groups is important, not just the predominant ones, such as the frontal thigh (quadriceps) muscles in runners. By working in a multidirectional resistive environment, better overall strength in the body or body part can be developed. No matter how or where you move, you are always working against the resistance of water.

• **Cross-Training.** Cross-training is important for the development of muscle symmetry. However, sports that are primarily one-sided require strength in other muscle groups to prevent overuse injuries. Examples of some unidirectional or primarily one-sided sports are golf, tennis and other racquet sports, and pitching in baseball.

• **Weight Loss.** When you raise the heart rate and metabolic rate through exertion, you start burning up those calories. This is like a trick mirror, though. Sometimes you lose weight, but most of the time you lose only body fat. Your clothes fit better and are looser, but your weight has not really changed. In fact, you may be increasing the lean muscle mass while you are losing body fat, and muscle weighs more than fat. It is better to judge your weight loss by the fit and feel of your clothes, rather than by the number of pounds lost.

• **Decrease in Cholesterol.** Many participants in water exercise report a noticeable drop in their "bad" cholesterol, known as high-density lipoprotein (HDL). This always makes their doctors smile!

• **Improved Bodily Functions.** Many people who take water exercise classes have reported significant improvement in their sleep patterns, as well as in their digestive systems. Exercise in the water can improve the overall efficiency of the body's systems.

CHOOSING YOUR EXERCISES

Part II presents a large collection of exercises that have been organized into beginner, intermediate, and advanced levels. Prior to beginning any exercise program, consult with your physician for the appropriateness of water exercise for your particular condition. If you are under the care of several doctors and one of them is a cardiologist, it is most important that you get this physician's clearance, even if another doctor has already cleared you. Each physician clears you medically for that condition for which he or she is treating you. Therefore, if a cardiologist is involved with your health care, please consult with him or her before undertaking an exercise program.

The following are suggested models for you to follow for fitness or rehabilitation.

Phase I: Beginner

Consider yourself a beginner if you have been sedentary for the majority of your life and have never participated in a consistent, structured exercise program. Also, if you have not been physically active in the past year, you should start at the beginner level. If you have been involved in an accident or are recovering from a recent surgery, start the program as a beginner. If you have any type of neuromuscular condition such as multiple sclerosis or parkinsonism, or if you have a rheumatic condition, begin at this level.

In the beginner phase, the goal is to establish a foundation of comfort with the water, improve the overall level of endurance, and increase the overall range of motion and flexibility of the body.

The beginner phase lasts about 2-4 weeks and proceeds as follows:

• Warm up. Walk forward, backward, and side-to-side for 10 minutes in chest-deep water.
• Proceed through the exercises in the beginner section in the sequence presented on page 158.

- Do one set of 15-20 repetitions for each exercise.
- End with a deep water workout (beginner phase) for 10-15 minutes nonstop.
- Rest or ice the area of injury after your workout.
- Exercise 3 days a week in the beginning.
- Allow a day of rest in between each workout.

Phase II: Intermediate

Consider yourself at the intermediate level if you have been fairly active physically in the past and have participated consistently in some activity that has an aerobic component 1-2 days a week. In other words, gardening does not count but walking does. You may move to the intermediate level when you have consistently participated at the beginner level and no longer find it challenging. Recreational or competitive athletes wishing to participate in a cross-training program can start at this level as long as they are not recovering from a significant injury.

At the intermediate level, you will be more challenged aerobically and will work against resistance in every exercise. Resistance to all lower extremity exercises is also increased through the use of surgical tubing. Exercises in this section are more demanding and require greater overall coordination, body control, and balance. The intermediate level focuses on building strength and coordination, whereas the beginner level focuses on range of motion and flexibility.

The intermediate phase lasts about 4-8 weeks and proceeds as follows:

- Warm up. Walk laps forward, backward, and side-to-side for 10 minutes.
- Proceed through the beginner exercises.
- Add intermediate exercises with resistance to your workout.
- Do two sets of 15 repetitions.
- End with a deep water workout for 20-30 minutes, nonstop.
- Use resistance either to the arms or legs, but not to both arms and legs in the deep water workout.
- Rest a day in between each workout.

Note. You may add a day of aerobic exercise only on the weekend. This can be bike riding, water jogging, or walking and should be 45-60 minutes in duration with little rest time.

Phase III: Advanced

The advanced level is appropriate for those individuals who have consistently participated at the intermediate level and no longer find it physically challenging. Also, competitive athletes or serious recreational athletes who have no injuries and are looking for a good cross-training program are appropriate for the advanced level. In this phase, the goal is to develop a high level of endurance, along with trunk strength and control. The exercises are designed to challenge and enhance trunk stability, balance, and overall coordination.

The advanced phase lasts about 8-12 weeks and proceeds as follows:

- Warm up. Walk laps as presented on page 87. Walk forward, backward, and side-to-side for 10 minutes using the advanced phase of the warm-up.
- Proceed through the intermediate level and advanced level sections. Start with the lower extremity workout, then go to the paddle and barbell exercises for the trunk, and the cord exercises for the trunk from the intermediate section. This should take at least 1 hour.
- Do three sets of 15 repetitions each.
- Finish with a 40-60 minute deep water workout. Use resistance with the arms and legs, or resistance with either the arms or legs, and increase the speed of your running.
- Incorporate some deep water workout advanced level exercises into your 40-60 minutes nonstop deep water jogging.

Note. Rest a day between workouts or do an extended (45-60 minutes) deep water workout on the day between the full workout sessions that involve the exercise and aerobic phases.

MAXIMIZING RESULTS

Design your program using those exercises that are most appropriate and enjoyable for you. One or two exercises may not be your favorites. The more you enjoy your workout, the more likely you will stay with the program long-term, and that is the ultimate goal: Exercise on a lifelong, consistent basis for better health and well-being. Exercising three to four times a week is a reasonable and productive goal. Make that commitment. When you reach your goal of recovery from an injury or a drop in weight, don't walk away from the program. To maintain those hard-earned results, some level of exercise must be included in your schedule three to four times a week from now on—in other words, a lifelong commitment.

As you progress through the program and incorporate harder exercises, you can drop the beginner level exercises. Your program will evolve with your progress and you should remain with a challenging but enjoyable series of exercises, anywhere from 60 minutes to 2 hours in duration. This will fluctuate with your schedule, but ideally, you will have designed a program that is accommodative.

The many benefits you will derive from a consistent exercise program are enduring and well worth your efforts!

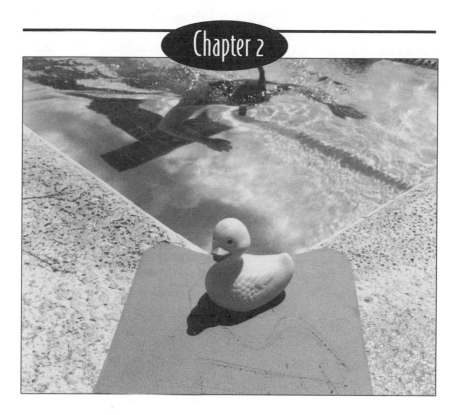

Chapter 2

Getting Prepared

Now that you have visited your doctor and have been cleared for water exercise, it is time to prepare yourself for exercise. In this chapter, you will learn how to select appropriate equipment and clothing to help you get the most out of your workout. You will also find advice on preparing the best environment for your workouts and tips on safety.

Just as a baseball player wouldn't step up to the plate without his helmet and bat, you shouldn't take to the water without appropriate clothing and equipment. A simple water exercise program might not require equipment, but this is not such a program. It is comprehensive, so you will need to take advantage of every possible tool to help maximize your efforts. The addition of the equipment used in this program enhances the strengthening component of the exercises by increasing resistance beyond that created by the movement of your body in the water. The addition of equipment will pay off in fitness and therapeutic results.

You wouldn't start a committed jogging or walking program without carefully selecting a good pair of shoes, would you? The same is true with water exercise. The equipment featured in this program is no more expensive than a good pair of athletic shoes and is just as important if you expect to get the most from your efforts. The equipment in the beginner phase adds moderate resistance and requires increased effort from the participant. However, the intermediate level incorporates exercises that require significantly more strength, balance, and overall control from the participant. The advanced phase continues with increased strength and balance demands, and requires coordination to complete the exercises successfully. You may find the beginner phase more to your liking, which is fine if that's where you are comfortable. In the event you do want to move past the entry or beginner level, you will find the how-to information and the specific equipment needs to advance your program in this chapter.

The following list represents the most basic equipment choices. You do not necessarily need each piece of equipment included here. You may find you want some or all of these, or you can substitute household items for some equipment. If you do decide to make water exercise a significant part of your fitness or therapeutic program, consider buying all of it, or perhaps buying it with a workout partner and sharing it.

• **Flotation Barbells.** The barbells come in various shapes and sizes. The triangular barbells from Aquajogger and the smaller, yellow barbells from Sprint have less resistance because of their surface size. The large blue barbells from Sprint offer maximum resistance. If you have significant shoulder or neck problems, you should opt for less resistance. Otherwise, choose the large blue barbells with maximum resistance.

• **Flotation Vests and Jogging Belts.** Flotation vests are made from flotation material that is custom-fitted according to body weight. They are expensive compared to the jogging belts and do not seem to offer any significant advantage. Aquajogger and Sprint, as well as some other manufacturers, offer jogging belts that come in small, medium, and large sizes. Both brands serve the same function and both are good products. Back patients are often more comfortable in the Sprint jogging belt because of its straight-back design, as opposed to the rounded humps on the Aquajogger belt. This rounded hump pitches the individual slightly forward in a vertical water posture. This position may be uncomfortable for some back patients, so they should use the

Sprint jogger belt or simply turn the Aquajogger belt upside-down with the humps facing downward instead of up toward the shoulders.

• **Hydro-Tone Boots and Barbells.** These are recommended only for those individuals in a fitness water exercise program. This equipment offers considerable resistance, which is too much in either the beginner or intermediate phases of rehabilitation, but could possibly be used in the advanced phase with proper supervision from a therapist.

• **Paddles.** The purchase of hand paddles is highly recommended. They are color-coded according to hand size (small, medium, large, and extra-large). You can go by your individual hand size or order larger or smaller paddles depending upon the amount of resistance you want to use with your program. When in doubt—order medium.

• **Aqua Steps (Reebok).** These are very popular with fitness enthusiasts and in water aerobic programs because they add another dimension to a fitness workout. These steps are the same equipment used for step aerobics on land.

• **Webbed Gloves.** These Neoprene gloves are excellent for individuals needing minimum resistance. Sprint gloves are useful for those with arthritic wrists, hands, or fingers. The Velcro closure at the wrist allows easy and pain-free access.

• **Goggles.** Purchase goggles to prevent chlorine irritation to the eyes if you will be doing any swimming.

• **Stretch Cords or Surgical Tubing.** This equipment is heavily used in therapeutic settings for graded or progressive muscle-strengthening programs. The cords or surgical tubing are color coded according to the amount of resistance of the industrialized rubber. They are available in retail outlets or medical supply houses. Two of the more popular brands are Life-Gym and Stretch-Cords (also Medi-Cords), the latter being manufactured by NZ Manufacturing. Their address is included in this chapter for your reference.

CHOOSING PROPER CLOTHING

When deciding what to wear in the water, consider the following guidelines.

• **Swimwear.** A typical   ; suit or loose-fitting shorts are sufficient. Something chlorine-resistant will last longer. If you tend to become chilled in water, consider a chlorine-resistant Lycra bodysuit, chlorine-resistant tights and a long-sleeved leotard, or a full bodysuit with long sleeves and long legs.

• **Shoes.** Aqua shoes or some type of light shoe are good for use in and out of the water. A light, inexpensive tennis shoe will suffice if you cannot find the aqua shoes, which are sometimes hard to find out of season. A light shoe adds significant traction and protects your feet in community shower areas. Most equipment and clothing are not expensive and are fairly easy to find. If you can't find the products locally, they may be available through mail order companies. (A list of manufacturers and clothing distributors appears on page 15).

If you are not in a position to purchase some of this equipment, you have several options. Birthdays, holidays, and special occasions are great times to present your equipment list to loved ones or friends. Why not get a friend to join you in your new fitness or rehabilitative venture and jointly buy and share some of the equipment? If that is not a viable option, simply substitute something else for the illustrated equipment. Large, plastic gallon milk jugs can substitute for hand barbells. Most public pools or community centers provide kickboards and long barbell floats upon request. Inexpensive, plastic saucers can be substituted for hand paddles. The stretch cords illustrated are available as Sports Cords or Life-Gym from large chain sporting goods stores. If you cannot find these, try a local medical supply house and ask for surgical tubing, Thera-Band or Thera-Tubing. Most individuals will do best with moderate-to-medium resistance. Men may need a bit more and should ask for medium-heavy, heavy, or heavy-plus resistance. Remember, buy the strength that allows you to do numerous repetitions in a controlled manner, not just one or two repetitions with faulty body mechanics.

EQUIPMENT AND CLOTHING MANUFACTURERS

Your first step should be to check with your local swimming supply store and other local merchants. Most carry the basic equipment. However, if you have difficulty finding just what you want, the following manufacturers carry all the supplies used in this water exercise program. Call them for a catalog or the location of the nearest merchant in your area.

Sprint Rothhammer
Box 5579
Santa Maria, CA 93456
800/235-2156
*(jogging belts, hand paddles,
hand dumbbells, kickboards,
floats, miscellaneous equipment,
including aqua shoes)*

NZ Manufacturing, Inc.
7405 S. 212 St., #125
Kent, WA 98032
800/886-6621
*(sports cords, stretch cords,
available for commercial
accounts)*

Hydro-Fit, Inc.
405 Lincoln St.
Eugene, OR 97401-2516
800/346-7295
*(cuff weights, hand dumbbells,
miscellaneous supplies, including
webbed gloves)*

Excel Sports Science
Box 1453
Eugene, OR 97440
*(Aquajogger belt, Aquajogger ankle
cuffs, dumbbells)*

Speedo
6040 Bandini Blvd.
Los Angeles, CA 90040
*(swimsuits and swim products,
resistive gloves, aqua shoes)*

Texas Swim Shop
11246 S. Post Oak Road, #102
Houston, TX 77035
713/723-0910
*(Sprint Rothhammer and NZ Manu-
facturing products: barbells, paddles,
stretch cords and belts, and
swimwear)*

PREPARING YOUR ENVIRONMENT

Now that you're ready to start your water exercise program, you need to find a pool that is convenient to you. Many of you will have a pool at your home, subdivision, or apartment complex. Community centers and local YMCAs or YWCAs are excellent aquatic resources, although they may be seasonal. Also, check with local high schools and colleges for their policies and fees for public use of the pool.

You want to choose a pool with both shallow and deep ends, ideally. Many apartment complex or home pools are designed with one depth, usually 4 to 5 feet; these are known as game pools. Fortunately, the workouts in the book can be modified for such pools, although the water jogging may have to be modified to include some light weightbearing. This will alter the intensity and overall cardiovascular output, but you can still derive strengthening, flexibility, and endurance benefits with the slightly slower pace.

ENSURING YOUR SAFETY

Work with a knowledgeable water exercise instructor or licensed thera-pist initially. Learning proper form, body mechanics, and precautions specific to an exercise is imperative to building a solid foundation. Any-one rehabilitating from injury or surgery is urged to get medical or li-censed supervision with the program.

Fitness enthusiasts are encouraged to join a water aerobics class, at first, to learn about heart rate monitoring and cardiovascular dos and don'ts. You will also learn aerobic or dance steps that will keep the water exercise program fresh, entertaining, and challenging. You want the pro-gram to be designed so that you will enjoy it over a long period of time.

For individuals needing a slower-paced program with good overall design and benefits, try the Arthritis Foundation Water Exercise Pro-gram. The instructors of this particular class are trained by the Arthritis Foundation and are knowledgeable about arthritis in general, joint pro-tection, and overall safety concerns specific to rheumatic conditions. In many cases, these classes may take individuals with other conditions in addition to arthritis, but this is determined by each class instructor.

Ask the instructor about his or her background and qualifications for teaching water exercise. Each instructor should be happy and willing to share that information and you certainly are entitled to it. You are trust-ing this individual with your health care needs, whether they are fitness-oriented or therapeutic in nature.

In addition to finding quality instruction, you should be aware of the following ways to ensure your safety.

Warm Up

It is important for you to prepare your body for a workout to avoid potential injury. Commit the first 10 minutes of your exercise routine to warming up in general by going through some easy multidirectional stretches. You may have a gentle stretching routine you already use that targets the large muscle groups of the body, including the front and back of the legs, the lower back, and the shoulders. Another good way to warm up is by walking forward across the pool in chest-deep water, then returning to the starting position by walking backward. This engages the entire body against resistance throughout the trunk, legs, and arms. Af-ter walking forward and backward for about 5 minutes, side-step across the pool and back, leading (stepping) with the right leg going across the pool and with the left leg on the return. By side-stepping across the pool, one works the inside and outside muscle groups on each leg, as well as the lateral or outer portions of the trunk on both sides of the body. The 10-minute walking in four directions increases the blood flow to all the muscles and raises the body temperature. Proceed through a series of gentle stretches from the head to the toes before increasing exertion by working against resistance. You always want to stretch a muscle that is warm to prevent injury or inflammation.

Temperature Settings

Most pools, especially community-based pools, are heated from 80 to 84 degrees Fahrenheit, which is comfortable and slightly cool. Anything below this range is intended more for competition and would not necessarily be appropriate or comfortable for the goals of fitness or rehabilitation. Therapeutic pools are heated from 86 to 90 degrees Fahrenheit and are ideal for arthritic, chronic pain, or post-surgical pain management conditions. Pools that teach young children and water-baby classes will have a warmer environment. In most cases, the therapeutic pool (86 to 90 degrees Fahrenheit) will meet most rehabilitative needs. If you are hypertensive, be very aware of the pool temperature and your comfort level. Avoid overexertion or overheating if you have a history of cardiac or hypertensive problems. The humidity outdoors or within the enclosed pool area will need to be monitored as well. Talk to the pool personnel about the temperature of the water and be aware of the environment.

If you have feelings of light-headedness or faintness, get to the side of the pool or the steps and let someone know what is happening. The same advice goes if you experience any tightness in the chest or left shoulder area. Always rest and make sure you are stable before returning to any level of exertion. If you are on several medications, talk to your doctor and discuss your plans for water exercise. Find out if there are any concerns regarding exercise and your current medications.

For fitness workouts, it is recommended that the temperature of the water be slightly cooler, about 80 to 84 degrees Fahrenheit. Because you will be engaging in an aerobic portion in your workout, your heart rate and body temperature will be elevated faster than for those working in a rehabilitative program. If you experience significant shortness of breath or labored breathing, take a few moments to rest, then continue your program at a pace that allows you to carry on conversation without losing your breath.

Drinking Water

The safest way for anyone to avoid overexertion in a water exercise program is to keep the body hydrated. Take some drinking water in a plastic container poolside so you can break every so often for a quick drink. Avoid glass containers at the pool! Water will keep the body temperature down and avoid any possibility of an accident. As pleasant as the pool can be, it is also deceptive. It allows so much more freedom of movement that we are unaware of other concerns, such as dehydration or overexertion. Play it safe when you enter the pool. Be aware of the water temperature, environmental humidity, and be sure to stay hydrated.

Overdoing It

Remember what was said about water's subtle deception? We are so thrilled with our newfound movement and movement without pain that once again we are distracted by the properties of water. Much of the body's weight is eliminated, and we have water's buoyancy to lift and support us. Exercising was never so easy! While water does offer much freedom, remember too that you are always working against resistance no matter how or where you move. If a little bit is good, is more better? No, not in this case. It is better to do a little less the first time you work out in the water. Even if you still have energy at the end of your workout, you should stop. You will be fatigued later, most likely, and have probably done more and moved more than you have in a long time; it was just easier in the water. It is best to get an idea of your limits in the first couple of workout sessions so you will know within what parameters you can safely and effectively exercise. You can always add to your workout as you gain in endurance, flexibility, and strength. Remember, Rome was not built in a day, and you cannot resurrect the body in one workout session.

Protecting Your Skin and Hair

Hundreds of chemical particles float in the water that can lodge themselves in our skin and hair. How do we protect ourselves from this chemical warfare? Follow the rules that you learned as a child. Shower before entering and after leaving the water—especially if you have sensitive skin. Baby oil or highly emollient lotions should be applied after exiting the pool and showering. This will prevent excessive drying of the skin and scalp and, hopefully, the development of any skin rashes. Wear open sandals in the warmer weather to enable your toes to dry out to prevent tinea pedis, or athlete's foot. The skin is an organ that requires nurturing and care just like any other part of the body. In the colder weather, use commercial foot powders in your shoes to prevent athlete's foot.

Chlorine can dry the scalp and make the hair brittle if you are in the water a great deal. Use a swim or shower cap and any good shampoo with conditioner after exiting the pool. Several shampoos available in retail stores strip the chlorine from the hair and are used widely by competitive swimmers. The more popular brands are Pert Plus and Ultra-Swim. Most of us can maintain the health of our hair and scalp with regular shampooing and weekly conditioning. Just as we need to be aware of hydrating the body during exertion, we must also hydrate the skin and hair to counteract the depleting property of chlorine and other pool chemicals.

Now that you've prepared yourself properly for water exercise, let's take a look at the exercises.

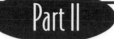

Water Exercises

Part II of *Water Exercise* introduces specific exercises through a step-by-step text with accompanying illustrations. The overall program design is broken down into a beginner level, covered in chapter 3; an intermediate level covered in chapter 4; and an advanced level covered in chapter 5. Chapter 6 introduces several deep water exercises that include the definitive text and exercise-specific illustrations.

The water exercise program was designed with beginner, intermediate, and advanced levels so each participant could start at his or her fitness level or rehabilitative stage and then progress safely into a more challenging stage at the appropriate time.

Equipment needs are defined in certain exercises. You may want to refer to chapter 2 for specific information on equipment. The addition of equipment really adds a whole new dimension to the overall program and its use is highly recommended. Water jogging should also be a part of your exercise routine. You can work on endurance, range of motion, flexibility, and strength simultaneously through water jogging. Once you get the hang of it, it is easy and comfortable. Get a partner to water jog with you and watch the time fly as you build a better and stronger body!

You will have some favorite exercises and some you can't stand! Go through them all once or twice and give them a try before you settle on your final program design. Remember to include some type of aerobic component, whether it is deep water jogging, jogging in shallower water, or doing some laps at the end of your workout.

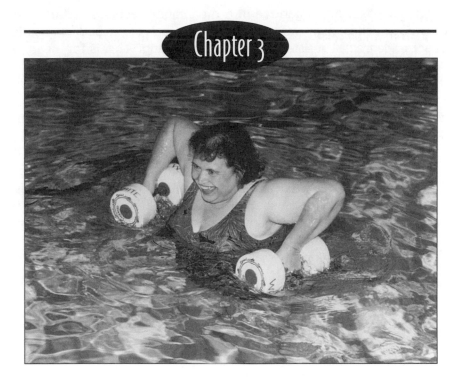

Chapter 3

Beginning Exercises

Chapter 3 introduces the beginner level of water exercises. In chapter 1, we defined the requirements for all three levels, beginner, intermediate, and advanced. The beginner level is for those who come from a sedentary background or who exercise occasionally but follow no structured program consistently. The beginner level is also appropriate for anyone starting in a therapeutic program following an injury, surgery, or period of inactivity due to pain or dysfunction.

Flexibility is strongly emphasized at this level. It is the most important component in a therapeutic program. Without flexibility, you will be unable to progress much further, and you will set yourself up for reinjury down the line.

The exercises are organized in a meaningful sequence. Start with a warm-up in chest-high water to engage as much of the body as possible in some degree of resistance prior to stretching. This is for safety, so don't skip your warm-up.

The majority of the exercises in the beginner section focus on flexibility or range of motion. There are a few that use some equipment for additional resistance and that focus on trunk strength and stability, and the ability to balance against additional resistance.

The first portion of the flexibility exercises in Chapter 3 focuses on the legs, especially the hips. The second portion includes the trunk-strengthening and resistive workout. The latter group of the beginner exercises can be done in the shallow end of the pool. All the other exercises are done in water chest high or above the waist. In this depth of water, you have to move against a greater degree of resistance to work the trunk. This will help you work as many of the muscle groups in the body as possible.

The exercises and the pages on which they appear follow.

Warm-Up Laps

Position: In chest-high water.

Description: Walk normally across the pool. When you reach the other side, walk *backward* across the water, returning to your original starting point. When you walk backward, keep your legs stiff and knees straight. Repeat several times, up to 8-10 minutes.

Note: This exercise may be difficult or uncomfortable when going backward. If it bothers you to walk stiff-legged when going backward, just walk normally. You may want to take smaller steps.

Precautions: Walking backward puts the lower back

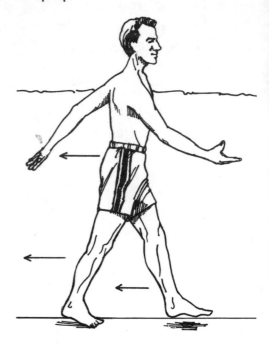

into extension, an area of weakness in many people. It also requires you to use hip extensors and hamstrings, the muscles in the back of the leg. If this exercise is bothersome initially, work up to it. Start out by walking forward only until you regain some flexibility and build your endurance. Do not walk backward if you have increased sharp lower back or leg pain. The back may not want to cooperate on this exercise.

No. 3.2   Sideways Walk

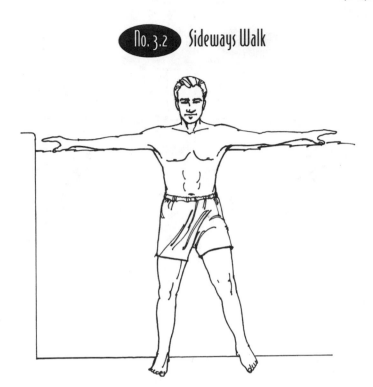

Position: Chest-high water, with the body turned sideways to the wall.

Description: Step sideways across the pool. Bring your feet together after each step and point them straight ahead. Do not let your foot roll out when you are leading the step. The stepping motion is initiated with the side of the hip. When you reach the other side, *do not* turn around—simply reverse your steps. This way, you lead with one leg going over and with the opposite leg coming back. If you turn around at the other side of the pool, you will be leading with the same leg both times. Repeat several times over and back across the pool.

Note: This exercise works each side of the trunk, hips, and lower extremities independently. If you tend to have problems on one side of the trunk or lower extremities, it is important to isolate and work each side of the body by moving in all directions—forward, backward, and side-to-side. This exercise works on overall flexibility.

Precautions: None.

No. 3.3 High Kicks

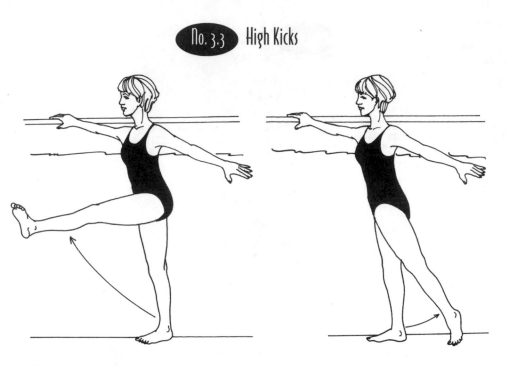

Position: Stand alongside the pool wall in chest-high water. Pull your foot up tight (as opposed to pointing it), and lift that leg up as high as it can comfortably go. The knee is locked and your opposite leg is straight with the heel down. The back should remain straight *no leaning forward or backward when kicking.* Heel flat!

Description: After kicking forward, push your leg backward in one continuous motion. It is not necessary to kick back very far. Again, your back stays straight—keep an upright posture. Continue with 20-30 repetitions on the same leg, then switch to the other leg.

Note: If you are unable to raise the leg very high due to hamstring tightness, that's okay. It is more important that you maintain an upright position. This exercise strengthens the quadriceps (front of the thigh) and hamstrings (back of the thigh), hips, and lower back.

Precautions: Do not extend your leg very far behind you. It is not necessary and can be uncomfortable. An extension of 12-18 inches is adequate.

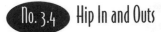

No. 3.4 Hip In and Outs

Position: Stand with your back against the pool wall in above-the-waist to chest-high water. Secure your arms or elbows along the edge of the pool wall for leverage.

Description: Raise your leg as high as is comfortably possible while keeping your back against the wall. Do not let your buttocks move off the wall. Pull the foot up tight—do not point the toe. Swing the leg out away from the body, then swing it back across the body in one continuous motion. Your other leg and knee are straight with the heel flat on the pool floor. Do 20-30 repetitions, then change legs.

Note: It is not necessary to swing your leg very far away from your body. It is more important to swing the leg across the whole body to get a full stretch on the hip and lower back. This exercise is for the inner and outer thighs and hips. We can all use this exercise!

Precautions: This exercise may be uncomfortable for acute lower back pain patients. If so, lower the leg and cross it over in front of the opposite leg and ankle and avoid straining the back or weaker hip. Remember to keep your back against the wall. This exercise should not be done if you have had a total hip replacement.

No. 3.5 Abdominal Press-Downs

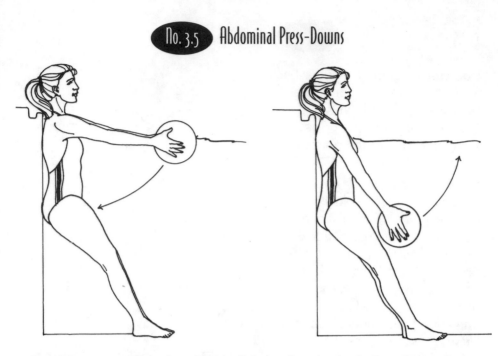

Equipment: Use a hand barbell, large floating barbell, or large plastic ball in the exercise.

Position: Lean back against the pool wall in above-the-waist to chest-high water. Spread the feet shoulder-width apart and place away from the wall about 12-18 inches. The barbell or large ball is held out at arm's length from the body, with the elbows locked and arms straight.

Description: Push the barbell or ball under the water and down to the hips, if possible. Slowly, release and repeat the exercise, *keeping the elbows locked*, 10-20 times or to your tolerance. You will feel this exercise immediately in the abdominals. Persevere, it gets easier.

Note: This is an excellent abdominal and trunk-strengthening exercise. It helps those flabby upper arms, as well. If you cannot get the float underwater, move to shallower water at first. To make the exercise more difficult, move to deeper water and/or put your feet together.

Precautions: Do not cheat on this exercise by leaning forward and using your body weight for leverage. *Keep that back against the wall!* This exercise uses both the abdominals and back extensors simultaneously. Move to shallower water or discontinue if this exercise increases lower back discomfort.

No. 3.6 Biceps Curl

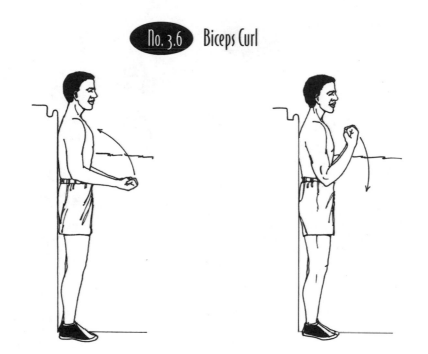

Position: Stand with your back against the pool wall in about chest-high water.

Description: The upper arm and elbow should be against the wall. Slowly raise the forearm and hand up in a curling motion toward the shoulder. Hold the position at the top of the movement, then slowly straighten the arm out completely. Do up to 20 repetitions, then switch arms. You may do the exercise for range of motion only, or you can add 1-5 lbs. of weight for more resistance.

Note: Be sure to keep the upper arm and elbow against the wall in this exercise. Also, completely lower the arm after each repetition in order to fully stretch the bicep, then repeat. You want to work the muscle through the entire range.

Precautions: If you are prone to elbow tendinitis or have arthritic problems in the elbows or shoulders, it is best to do this exercise with little or no weight (1-3 lbs. maximum). Concentrate primarily on going through the full range of motion. Using heavy wrist weights can easily overload or aggravate joint or tendon inflammation.

No. 3.7   Chest Flys

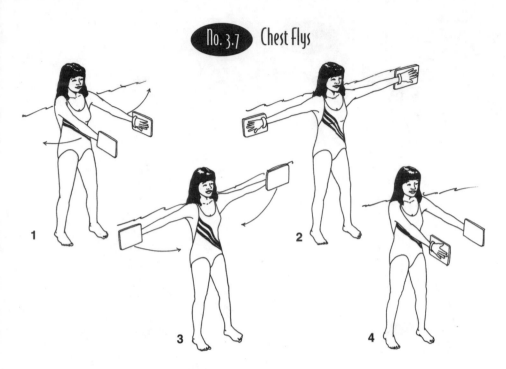

Equipment: Use your hand paddles with this exercise.

Position: Stand in above-the-waist to chest-high water, feet shoulder-width apart and pointing straight ahead. Hand paddles should be secured with the palms facing outward and the elbows locked.

Description: Slowly push your arms back and away from you with the paddles just under the surface of the water. After your arms are directly out to your sides, flip the paddles over so the palms are coming together as you push the water forward. Again, turn the palms over facing away from each other and push straightened arms back and away. Repeat 20-30 times.

Note: This exercise tends to knock people off balance when they flip the paddles over and push the water forward. Tighten the lower back and buttocks and lean into the exercise slightly at the hips when pushing the hands forward and together. This is an excellent upper back and posture exercise.

Precautions: If you are having trouble keeping your balance, move to shallower water for better leverage, or widen your stance.

No. 3.8 Shoulder Press-Downs

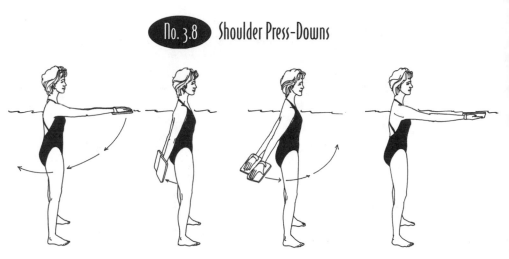

Equipment: Use your hand paddles with this exercise.

Position: Stand in chest-high water. Your feet are spread shoulder-width apart with the knees locked. Hold your arms in front of your body with your elbows locked and palms facing down.

Description: Press your arms and hands down toward the hips, keeping them close to your body. When your hands and arms are parallel with the hips, flip the hands over and, keeping elbows locked, push toward the water's surface. Repeat 20-30 times, or to your tolerance. Add hand paddles with this exercise for more resistance.

Note: If you tend to lose your balance on this exercise, move to slightly shallower water. If you need the exercise to be more challenging, use larger hand paddles or move into deeper water. Also, to make this exercise harder, put the feet together; this requires more trunk strength and stabilization.

Precautions: This exercise should not be that difficult. Follow the above modifications if necessary and be sure you have a wide base of support (feet shoulder-width apart). This is all about balance and learning to adjust when your center of gravity changes.

No. 3.9 Internal and External Shoulder Rotation

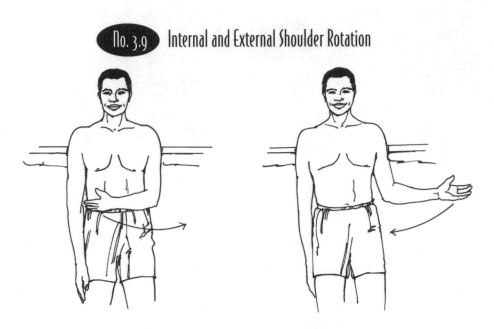

Position: Lean back against the wall in chest-high water. Tuck your upper arms and elbows snugly against your sides.

Description: Cup your hands and fingers; place your hands over your abdomen. With your elbows tucked against your sides, press your forearm back toward the wall. Reverse and bring your lower arm back over the abdomen. Do 10-20 repetitions. Both arms can be done together or one arm at a time.

Note: The key to this shoulder exercise is keeping the upper arm and elbow pressed in against your side. This exercise rotates the upper arm (humerus) in the shoulder joint. With a shoulder injury, or "frozen shoulder," this motion is usually markedly restricted or lost altogether if the area is not exercised.

Precautions: None.

No. 3.10 Trunk Twists

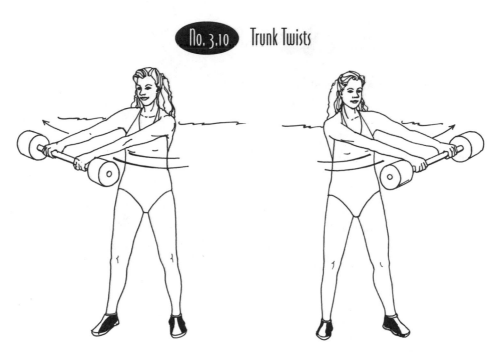

Equipment: Use a kickboard or large floating barbell with this exercise.

Position: This exercise can be done in above-the-waist to chest-high water.

Description: Using a floating barbell (or a kickboard held at each end), slowly twist from side to side as far as you can possibly go. The feet should be shoulder-width apart and pointing straight ahead. As you twist from side to side, the heels should stay flat to allow for more of a stretch.

Note: This is a flexibility exercise and should be done in a smooth, controlled fashion. To get maximum benefits, do the exercise slowly and concentrate on stretching. Arms should be held as stiff as possible.

Precautions: This exercise should not be done in a rushed motion. Full trunk rotation may be uncomfortable for people suffering from chronic or acute lower back pain. Shorten the twisting motion or avoid altogether if this causes increased discomfort.

No. 3.11   Marching in Place

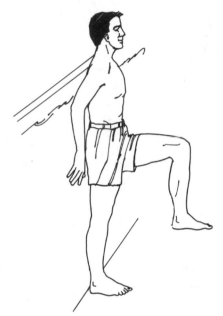

Position: Stand in chest-high water with your back flat and fully supported against the pool wall. Rest hands lightly against the pool wall.

Description: While keeping the back flat against the wall, bend each knee and hip up as high as you comfortably can, alternating the legs in a marching motion. The back and shoulders remain flat against the wall as much as possible. Avoid leaning forward at the hips. Complete up to 20 repetitions on each leg.

Note: By keeping your back against the wall, you avoid leaning into flexion of the trunk. This position causes cumulative wear and tear on the lower back. You also stretch the hamstrings, hips, and lower back with this exercise.

Precautions: If you have had a total hip replacement within the past 10 weeks, DO NOT flex the hip more than 90 degrees. In the early stages following hip surgery, avoid any motion above a 90-degree angle to ensure safety in regard to the prosthesis.

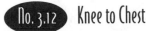 Knee to Chest

Position: Stand in chest-high water with your back flat and fully supported against the pool wall.

Description: While keeping the back completely flat against the wall, bend the knee up toward the chest. Pull the knee in against the chest and hold it there for 5-10 seconds before lowering it. Complete 5-10 repetitions on the same leg, then switch and repeat the stretch on the other side, 5-10 times. Remember to keep the back and shoulders as flat against the wall as possible.

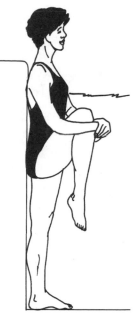

Note: This is an excellent lower back and hip stretch. By performing this move in chest-high or slightly lower water, the load or pressure on the vertebrae and discs of the spine is reduced about 70%.

Precautions: This is a low back stretch. DO NOT do this stretch if you have had hip replacement surgery!

No. 3.13   Barbell Push-Pulls

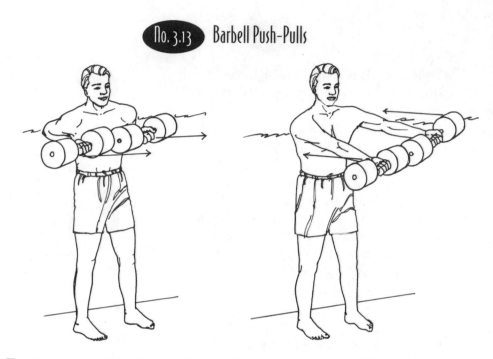

Equipment: Use the hand barbells or large plastic milk jugs in this exercise.

Position: Stand in water above the waist to shoulder high. Spread your feet shoulder-width apart and point them straight ahead. Grasp each dumbbell with your palms facing up.

Description: Push the barbells forward and out from your body and then pull them back in. Legs remain straight with the knees locked. Repeat 20-30 times at a fast pace—no resting in between repetitions! You may either alternate your arms or do them at the same time.

Note: This exercise is for upper back posture. Doing the exercise fast creates more turbulence in the water, thus more resistance. By repeating as many as possible without resting, you build endurance and upper body strength.

Precautions: If possible, do both arms together. However, if this causes premature fatigue, start by alternating the arms. From there pick up your pace, then increase your repetitions. When you get stronger, you can try doing the exercise for a certain time, i.e. 30 seconds, 1 minute, and so on without stopping and resting.

No. 3.14   Gorilla Press-Downs

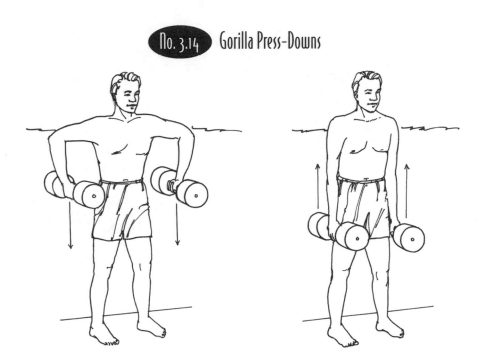

Equipment: Use the hand barbells or large plastic milk jugs in this exercise.

Position: Stand in water approximately chest high. Point your feet straight ahead, shoulder-width apart. Place the dumbbells under your armpits. Looks just like a monkey scratching under his arm!

Description: Press the dumbbells down until your arms are fully extended. Slowly release and repeat 10-20 times, to your tolerance.

Note: This is a posture exercise for the upper back. There is some strengthening benefit, but this primarily corrects poor posture.

Precautions: None. This exercise is easy. Some individuals may notice upper back or shoulder tightness, due to postural dysfunction. This is great for the rounded-shoulder posture that your mother referred to as "slumping"!

No. 3.15 Bird

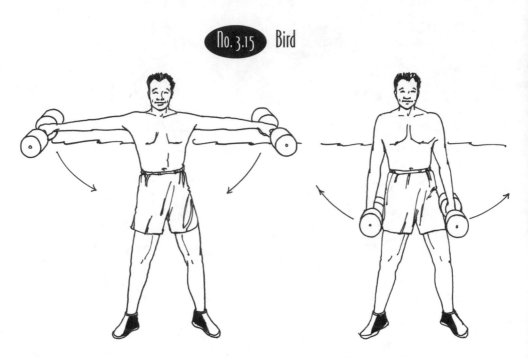

Equipment: Use the hand barbells or large plastic milk jugs.

Position: Stand in water above the waist to chest high. Extend your arms and elbows straight out at shoulder level, with the palms facing down. Feet are shoulder-width apart.

Description: Push arms straight down to the sides, then relax slowly. Repeat 10-20 times, doing both arms simultaneously.

Note: Push both arms down at the same time. If this is difficult, move to shallower water. Likewise, to increase the difficulty, move to deeper water and/or put the feet together. This exercise strengthens the upper and middle back and shoulders.

Precautions: None. Follow the previous modifications as needed.

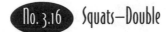 **Squats—Double**

Position: 'Face the pool wall in waist-high water. Feet are pointing straight ahead, not pointing outward, and placed 4 in. to 6 in. apart.

Description: Squat down as far as you can comfortably go, while keeping your *heels down*. If you reach a point where your heels begin to pull up from the pool floor, do not go any further; this will be your maximum point of flexion.

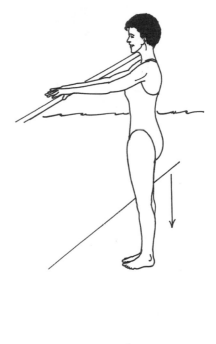

Note: You do not want to do this exercise with the heels off the pool floor, because that would really affect the efficiency of the exercise. If this exercise is too easy, move away from the wall into the middle of the pool. Now you are working on balance as well as lower extremity strength and flexibility. Do this exercise slowly. Doing it quickly uses momentum rather than strength and it isn't as effective overall. In fact, it's cheating.

Precautions: This exercise may be bothersome for individuals with arthritic knees or any type of patellar (kneecap) problem. Those individuals should move to slightly deeper (above the waist) water and do squats to a 45-degree angle versus a deep knee bend. Do not do this exercise if it is too painful.

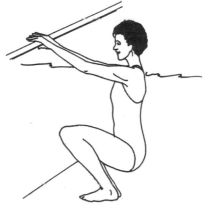

No. 3.17   Squats—Single

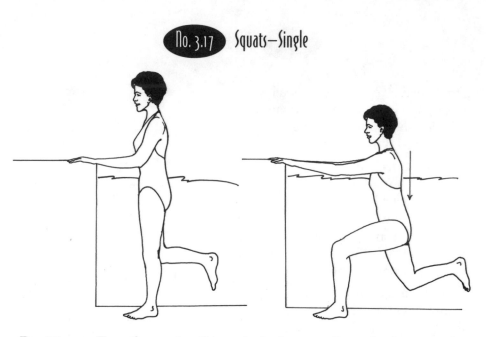

Position: Face the pool wall in waist-high water. Point the feet straight ahead, not pointing outward. The feet are 4 in. to 6 in. apart.

Description: This exercise is exactly like the two-legged squats, except it is done with one leg. This is excellent for strengthening a weak hip, knee, or ankle. The uninvolved leg is behind you and is either non-weightbearing or lightly touching the pool floor to help with balance. Squat down as far as you can comfortably go, while keeping the heel down. If you reach a point where your heel begins to pull up from the pool floor, do not go any further; this will be your maximum point of flexion.

Note: You do not want to do this exercise with the heel off the pool floor, as that would negate the efficiency of the exercise. Also, if this exercise is too easy, move away from the wall into the middle of the pool. Now you will be working on balance as well as lower extremity strength and flexibility. Do this exercise slowly. If you do it too quickly, you use momentum rather than strength.

Precautions: This exercise may be bothersome for individuals with arthritic knees or any type of patellar (kneecap) problems. It is suggested that those individuals move to slightly deeper (above the waist) water and do squats to a 45-degree angle versus a deep knee bend. Do not do this exercise if it is too painful.

No. 3.18   Ankle Inversion

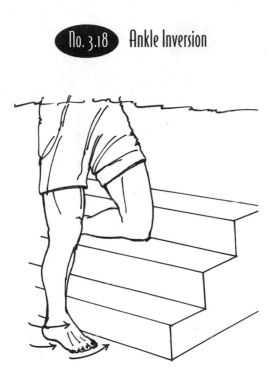

Position: Stand next to the pool wall or sit on the pool steps in shallow water. Place the inside of the foot (big toe side) next to the wall.

Description: Press the inside of the foot against the wall. Hold the contraction to the count of "10." Relax 5 seconds, then repeat the motion, pressing the inside of the foot into the wall. Hold to a count of "10" and relax. Repeat 10-20 times and switch to the opposite ankle.

Note: This exercise is done more effectively with the knee flexed because it isolates the ankle. This allows less chance for substitution or compensation for the weak ankle by stronger muscle groups. All repetitions should be done on one ankle before switching to the other; this builds strength and endurance.

Precautions: None.

Ankle Eversion

Position: Stand next to the pool wall or sit on the pool steps in shallow water. Place the outside of the foot (side with the little toe) next to the wall. Flex the knee to isolate the ankle movements.

Description: Press the lateral side (little toe) into the side of the pool wall or step and hold the contraction to the count of "10." Relax 5 seconds and repeat, pressing the side of the foot with the little toe into the wall. Hold to a count of "10" and relax. Repeat 10-20 times, or to your tolerance. Repeat on opposite ankle.

Note: This exercise is best done with the knee flexed to isolate the ankle. If the exercise is done with a

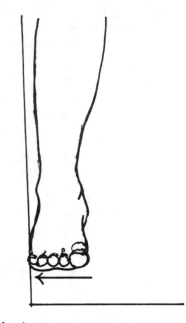

straight leg, there is a greater chance of substitution or compensation for ankle weakness by stronger muscles. Do all repetitions on one ankle before switching to the other ankle.

Precautions: None.

Hip Abduction Facing Wall

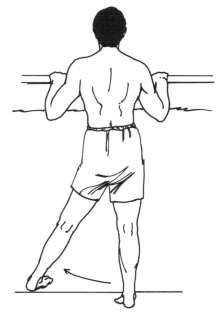

Position: Face the wall in above-the-waist to chest-high water. Stand with the feet 6 inches apart and pointing straight ahead.

Description: Raise the leg out to the side with the toe turned inward (pigeon-toed). *Keep the back straight!* No bending of the trunk to try to get the leg higher. The leg will only go to about a 45-degree angle. Be sure you are not turning your trunk slightly to help raise the leg. This is cheating and will not help your body! Repeat 20 times on one side, then switch legs.

Note: Critical! Keep the leg pigeon-toed so that the correct muscle group is isolated and strengthened. If you have some trunk inflexibility and tightness, your body will try to work around this! The back stays straight—no bending or turning of the trunk!

Precautions: If this causes hip or back pain, most likely you are substituting (fancy word for cheating). Check and make sure your back is straight and there is no rotation of the trunk. The leg comes directly out to the side. There should be no pain (though there may be some discomfort) if this exercise is done right.

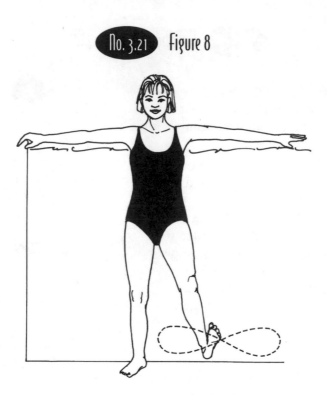

No. 3.21   Figure 8

Position: This exercise may be done standing along the pool wall in 3 to 4 feet of water or sitting down on the pool steps.

Description: Slowly trace a figure 8 in the water. It may be done vertically—an up-and-down motion, or horizontally—tracing the figure 8 in a side-to-side motion.

Note: This is a good exercise to do if you find the other hip exercises too aggressive.

Precautions: This exercise should not be difficult or uncomfortable. It can be done by total hip replacement patients in the vertical position only.

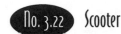 Scooter

Equipment: Use a large floating barbell with this exercise.

Position: Position the floating barbell just under your bottom and sit on it. You should be in the shallow end of the pool where your feet are flat on the ground. Grasp hands together in front of you. You should be sitting as though you are in a chair—hips and knees at about a 90-degree angle.

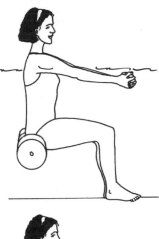

Description: Remember, your hands are clasped together in front of you. Stretch your leg out in front of you and touch down with the heel. Pull yourself forward using your heel and leg, until the leg is flexed (bent) under you and you are on the ball of the foot. Now, stretch the other leg all the way out in front of you and touch down with the heel. Repeat all the way across the pool, then reverse and go backward across the pool. To reverse, straighten the leg by pushing back with your toes. Repeat across the pool, returning to your original starting point. When crossing the pool, you pull yourself forward with your heel. To reverse, you push yourself backward by pushing off the ball of the foot.

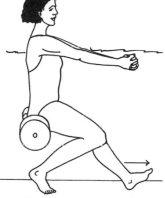

Note: An important aspect of this exercise is getting a full stretch on the muscles, going forward and backward.

Precautions: This exercise requires some balance. If possible, try it with your hands clasped in front of you to really isolate the legs. Going across the pool will be harder than coming back because the hamstrings (back of the thigh) are weaker in most people, and that is the muscle you will be using.

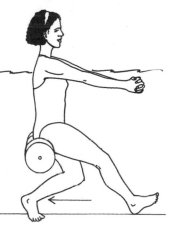

No. 3.23   Wrist Curls

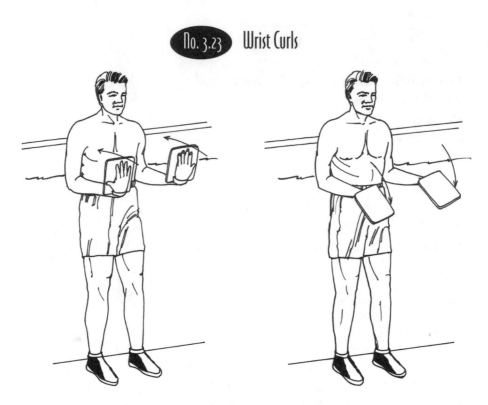

Position: Stand in chest-high water with the back flat and fully supported against the wall. Place the upper arms and elbows against the wall. Bend the elbows to a 90-degree angle with palms facing up.

Description: Bend both wrists in toward the body then extend them out and away. For additional resistance, use webbed gloves or hand paddles. Be sure to bend (flex) the wrists in as far as possible, then extend hands out and away as far as possible, too. Repeat 10-20 times or to tolerance.

Note: This exercise works the wrist flexors and extensors, the muscles of the forearm. It is good for any wrist or hand injuries, especially if you were casted. Also, if there is any swelling or injury to the shoulder, it is important to work the elbow and wrist in addition to the shoulder.

Precautions: None. Additional resistance can be added with webbed gloves or paddles. Avoid this if you have or are prone to tendinitis of the wrists or elbows.

No. 3.24   Adductor Squeezes

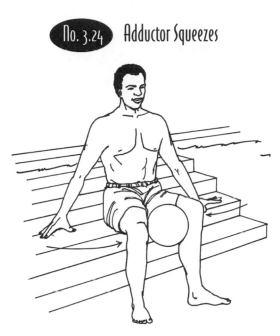

Equipment: Use a medium-sized rubber or plastic ball with this exercise.

Position: Sit on the pool steps. If there are no steps, lean against the pool wall in shallow water, with the knees and hips bent at a 90-degree angle, as if sitting in a chair. The back is supported completely by the wall and the feet are flat.

Description: Place a medium-sized rubber or plastic ball between your knees. Keep your feet flat and your knees and hips bent. Squeeze the ball as hard as you can and hold it for 5-10 seconds. Release and repeat, holding the position for 5-10 seconds. Repeat up to 20 times and relax.

Note: This exercise works the inner thighs and hips. Do this exercise to strengthen your inner thigh muscles, the adductors, if you have had any knee or hip surgery.

Precautions: None. Remember, if you have had hip surgery, do not go above 90 degrees of hip flexion.

No. 3.25   Unloading the Spine

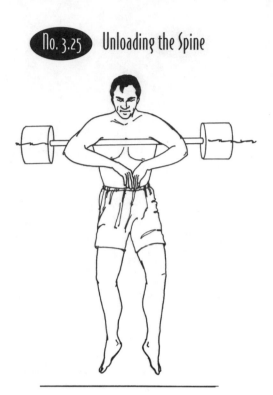

Equipment: Use a large floating barbell, hand barbells, or a kickboard with this exercise.

Position: You can do this in deep or chest-high water. Place barbell under your arms and lean your body weight slightly forward onto the barbell.

Description: Raise your legs off the pool floor either in front or behind you. Obviously, if you are in deeper water, you will just hang from the barbell. However, not everyone is comfortable in the deep end. You can hang from the barbell and touch your heels on the pool bottom in front of you. Hang anywhere from 5 to 15 minutes.

Note: This exercise opens up the space between the vertebrae of the spine and takes pressure off the discs and nerve roots. The important thing is to get the body weight completely off the legs. This allows the back to fully stretch and "unload" pressure off the discs.

Precautions: None. This exercise is a great way to manage your back pain.

No. 3.26 Heel Rock and Rolls

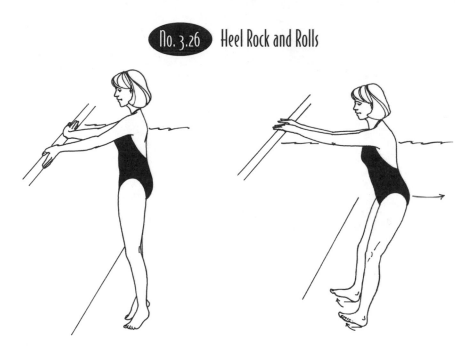

Position: Face the pool wall in chest-high water. The feet are point-ing straight ahead and are 4 inches apart.

Description: Raise up as far as possible on the toes, then lean back and rock on the heels, toes up. Your knees are locked. Repeat 20-30 times to your tolerance—up on the toes, then roll back on the heels.

Note: Stand fairly close to the wall so that when you rock back onto your heels, you will not be straining with the lower back. When you raise up on your toes, you can rock the hips in slightly (knees stay locked) and then rock the hips back when you roll back onto your heels. This motion is a great range-of-motion exercise for the lower back.

Precautions: None.

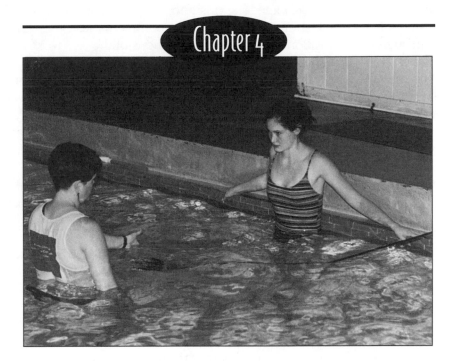

Intermediate Exercises

While chapter 3 focused primarily on the development of overall flexibility, chapter 4 focuses on the development of strength. All the exercises in this chapter work with some type of additional resistance or require increased or sustained endurance to successfully complete the exercise. Once you have improved your overall flexibility, the goal of the beginner level exercises, you can move safely to a more challenging stage of your rehabilitative or fitness program.

The latter portion of the intermediate exercises involves jumping or balancing on one leg. This requires sustained strength or endurance. If you do not have the degree of endurance or strength needed to balance in the specified posture, you will not be able to complete the exercise.

In all intermediate level exercises, position is very important. You will be using a lot of trunk strength and control to complete these exercises. Carefully read the position and description portions of the text to ensure proper technique and safety.

You might want to refer back to chapter 2 on equipment. A company called NZ Manufacturing (see chapter 2) carries the stretch cords you will need. It has kits that are made specifically for the back, leg, or other areas. They also sell handles and padded ankle attachments to go with the cords. The cords are color coded, with each color designating a certain level of resistance. These levels go from light to heavy duty. A chart defines each color and its corresponding level; a sales representative or therapist can suggest the appropriate grade of resistance for you. Another product, known as Thera-Tubing, is used in many rehabilitation clinics. It is also color-coded for different levels of resistance. Life-Gym is a kit that is available in many large sporting goods stores around the country, as well as at some medical supply stores. Check under "physical therapy equipment" in your local Yellow Pages for information on this line of equipment. The stretch cords and Life-Gym come with various accessories that are very useful. You also can use them for land-based exercises.

Not everyone will want, or need, strength training as part of an exercise or therapeutic program. Some but not all of my patients go through the intermediate exercises. It depends on their needs and overall therapy goals. If you are in a therapeutic program, ask your therapist to tell you which exercises in this section are appropriate for you in your personal rehabilitation.

As far as fitness is concerned, a strengthening portion is advisable for your overall fitness program, as is an aerobic portion. It's up to you how much emphasis you want to put on the strengthening phase of your fitness workout. If you want a strong emphasis on resistive training, purchase one of the kits described earlier. It can be used on land as well, which makes it attractive for cross-training.

The exercises and the pages on which they appear follow.

No. 4.1   Alternate Press-Downs

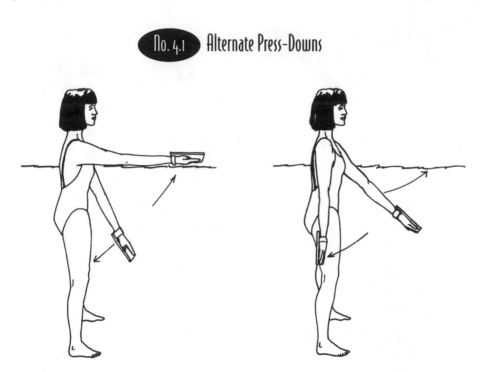

Equipment: Use the hand paddles with this exercise for increased resistance.

Position: Stand with a wide base of support (feet shoulder-width apart) with the legs straight and the knees locked. One arm will be held straight out in front of the body, elbow locked, palm facing downward. Hold the other arm down at the hip, elbow locked, palm facing upward.

Description: Press the upper arm downward while lifting the lower arm toward the surface of the water. This creates a push-pull type of movement. Continue alternating the arms while keeping the elbows locked. Repeat 20-30 times, or to your tolerance.

Note: It is important to have a wide base of support and to keep the arms close to the sides. The further the arms are from the sides of the body, the more resistance on the lower back, shoulder, and elbow joints.

Precautions: If this creates too much strain on the lower back, widen your base of support or move to shallower water. This exercise isolates each side of the body and will create a slight rotation of the spine at the same time. This is great for loosening up a stiff back! Anybody out there have a stiff back? Several million people, it's estimated!

No. 4.2 The Runner

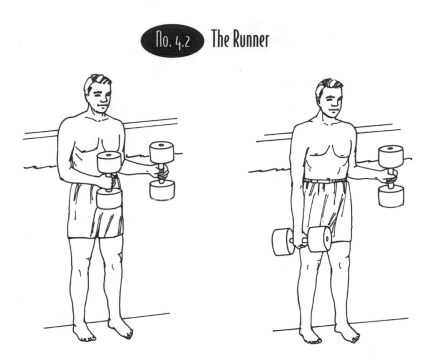

Equipment: Use the hand barbells or large milk jugs with this exercise.

Position: Stand in water about chest high. Grasp dumbbells with elbows bent at a 90-degree angle and pressing against the ribs.

Description: Push the dumbbells down until the arm is straight and the elbow is locked. Keep the arm close to the side for better control. Relax and repeat 10-20 times, to your tolerance. Switch arms and repeat.

Note: It is important that you start at a 90-degree angle and push down until your arm is straight and your elbow is locked. Adjust your position depth-wise so that you can determine the resistance. For more resistance, move into deeper water, for less, move into shallow water.

Precautions: None. This exercise should pose no problems; you may become aware of specific muscle (triceps) weakness. Running was never so easy! The arms mimic a sprinter's form in this exercise.

No. 4.3 Wall Push-Ups

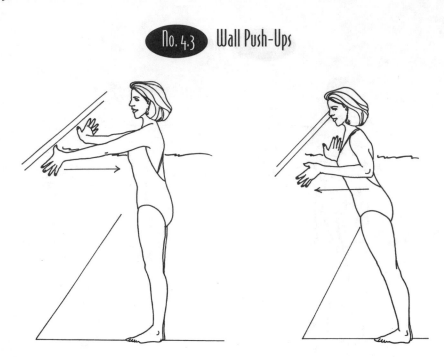

Position: Stand in water above the waist to chest high. Place your arms on the side of the pool in front of the shoulders. Your elbows are pointing outward on this exercise.

Description: Stand an arm's length away from the wall. Your feet are shoulder-width apart. Lean the body forward, supporting it on the hands as you approach the wall. The trunk is straight—do not bend at the hips. Straighten your arms back to their fully extended position and repeat. If you can keep the heels down, do so, for this will stretch the ankles. If not, try to keep most of the foot on the ground as you lean forward. Repeat 10-20 times, or to your tolerance.

Note: This exercise works the arms and the upper back and chest. It is good for any upper extremity injury.

Precautions: None. If this exercise causes discomfort in the shoulders or neck, move in closer to the wall so that the arms are not fully extended.

No. 4.4   Washboard

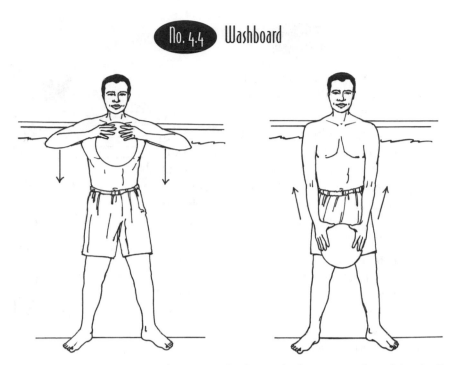

Equipment: Use a medium-sized plastic ball or your hand barbells with this exercise.

Position: Stand in water above the waist to chest high. The back is flat and fully supported against the wall. Feet are shoulder-width apart and flat on the ground.

Description: Place a medium-sized plastic or rubber ball at chest level. Pretend the ball is a clock and place the hands at the 10 and 2 o'clock positions. Push the ball straight down toward the hips and release up slowly. Keep the ball close to the body and the back flat against the wall. The elbows are locked and straight. Repeat 20-30 times, or to tolerance.

Note: This exercise works the upper back, chest, and arms. By keeping the back flat against the wall, you use upper body and arm strength. Also, keeping your back against the wall supports and stabilizes the trunk and prevents you from bending forward at the hips. Try to avoid that forward-flexed position of the trunk whenever you can.

Precautions: If this exercise causes back, neck, or shoulder discomfort, move to shallower water to lessen the resistance. If discomfort persists, avoid this exercise altogether. It may be uncomfortable for those with neck conditions. Listen to your body!

No. 4.5 Upright Rows With Cords

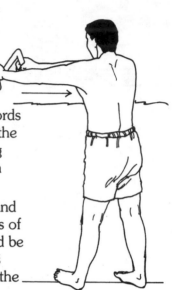

Equipment: Use stretch cords or surgical tubing with this exercise.

Position: Secure the cords to a fixed and stable object, such as a handrail or pool ladder in the shallow end of the pool. Slowly back up while holding the cords with your arms out straight. Back away until the cords are taut. Your feet should be pointing straight ahead, with the legs shoulder-width apart for leverage.

Description: With the arms outstretched and cords taut, slowly pull the cords in to the sides of your body at a chest-high level. Elbows should be pointing back when you are finished with this move. Now, slowly release the cords back to the original starting position, which is arms outstretched in front of you with the cords taut. Do 10-20 repetitions, according to your tolerance.

Note: It is important this exercise be done with control—not at a hurried pace. At a slow, controlled pace, the exercise maximizes the targeted muscles. A wide stance lends support and helps you keep your balance.

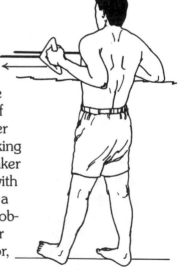

Precautions: This is a demanding exercise that requires strength, balance, and control. If you can't keep your heels down, step in closer until you are able to stay balanced while working against resistance. Some individuals with weaker upper backs may have to start this exercise with their arms slightly bent until they progress to a point where balance and control are not a problem. Remember, everyone works at his or her own pace—don't compete with your neighbor, just proceed carefully for the best results and safety's sake.

No. 4.6 Punches With Cords

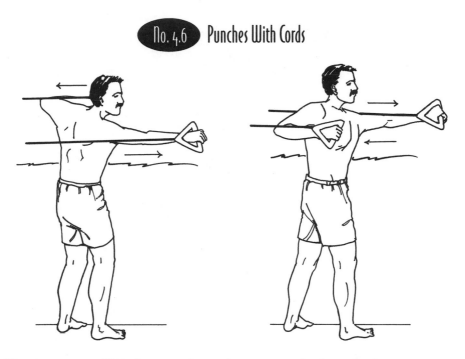

Equipment: Use the stretch cords or surgical tubing in this exercise.

Position: Secure the cords to a fixed and stable object, such as a hand-rail or pool ladder in the shallow end of the pool. Grab the cord handles and slowly walk away, with your back turned to the cord attachment. Handles should be placed directly in front of your shoulders and the cords should be taut. Your feet are pointing straight ahead and are shoulder-width apart.

Description: Push one arm straight ahead, as if throwing a punch, then alternate with the other arm. Punch forward until the arm is fully extended, then release and slowly return to the original starting position. Feet stay flat on the ground. This enables the upper trunk/body to rotate about a fixed (stationary) pelvis; keep hips still. The rotation comes from the waist up. Repeat 10-20 times, according to your tolerance.

Note: You may find yourself leaning in as you "throw punches." That's fine as long as the majority of the work is done by the upper back and arm. Remember, the pelvis is stationary; all the rotation is above the waist.

Precautions: Be sure to "throw punches" straight ahead, with the arm close to the body. If you punch out to the side, or away from the trunk of the body, you increase stress on the shoulder joint, neck, and lower back, and that should be avoided.

No. 4.7 Side-Swipes With Paddle

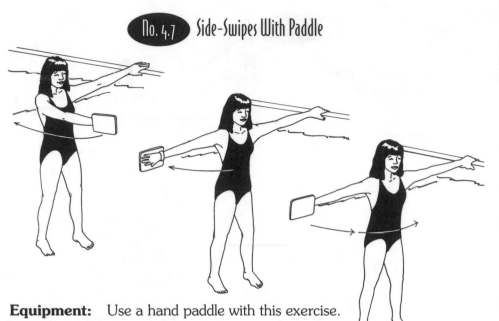

Equipment: Use a hand paddle with this exercise.

Position: Stand in water above the waist to chest high. Stand sideways to the pool wall with your left arm directly out to the side, fully extended with the elbow locked. Grasp the side of the pool for support. Place the paddle on the right hand with the palm facing away from the wall. Place your feet shoulder-width apart.

Description: While holding on to the side with your left arm straightened, sweep the right hand across and away from the body with the palm turned out. When you reach your end range, turn the paddle over so that the palm is turned in. Now, sweep the arm forward and across the body toward the pool wall. Repeat 10-20 times, then switch the paddle to the other hand and repeat.

Note: This exercise requires the full use of the trunk and arms. You will definitely feel this exercise, especially if you have trunk weakness. Be sure you can do all the other hand paddle exercises before you move to this one. It is important to keep the arm that is holding on to the wall fully extended with the elbow locked.

Precautions: If this exercise pulls you off your feet or you feel increased back pain, move to shallower water for better support and leverage. If you are unable to do it without pain, discontinue and concentrate on the other hand paddle exercises a bit longer.

No. 4.8 Sideways Cross-Over With Cords

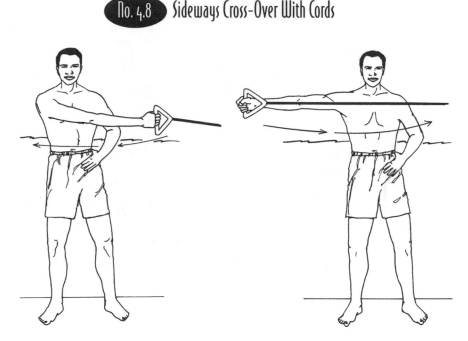

Equipment: Use the stretch cords or surgical tubing with this exercise.

Position: Secure the cords to a fixed and stable object, such as a handrail or pool ladder in the shallow end of the pool.

Description: Step away from the cords sideways, until your right arm is fully extended across your chest; your left side is closest to the cords. Spread your feet shoulder-width apart for leverage. Place your left hand on your left hip for additional support. With the right elbow locked, pull the cord out and across your body to the right side. Then slowly release and return to the starting position. Repeat 10-20 times, to your tolerance. Now switch sides so that your right side is closest to the cords, and your left arm is fully extended across your chest with the elbow locked. Pull the cord out and across your body to the left side and return to the starting position. Repeat to your tolerance.

Note: This is a very challenging exercise and requires good trunk strength. You may find one side to be stronger or weaker. Adjust the exercise according to the strength of each side by moving in closer or stepping further out.

Precautions: Do not do this exercise if it causes increased pain.

No. 4.9 Biceps Curl

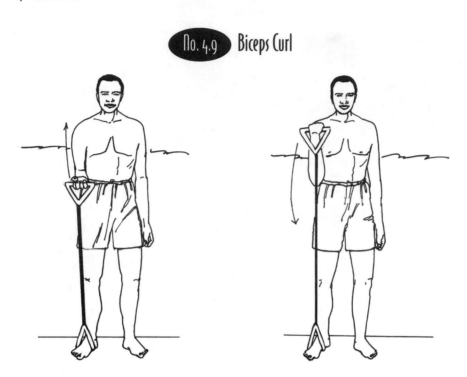

Position: Stand in chest-high water. You may use the pool wall for added back support, or work the back by doing this exercise away from the wall. Stand with your feet shoulder-width apart.

Description: Anchor the resistive tubing or band under the foot on the same side of your body. Your arm should be fully extended in the starting position. Slowly curl the forearm and wrist up toward the shoulder as far as you can. Hold that muscle contraction 3 seconds, then slowly release the arm down into the fully extended position. Repeat up to 20 repetitions then switch to the other arm. The arm should start directly in front of the hip and end near the shoulder joint. Keep your elbows tucked tightly against your rib cage.

Note: To make this exercise harder, do both arms at the same time, or anchor the tubing on a bar or stick, to create a barbell. *Please*, if you do the double curl, make sure you protect your back by slightly bending the knees, and tightening your abdominals and lower back.

Precautions: You may want to skip this exercise if you have any neck problems or pain. Also, be careful with this exercise if you have elbow joint pain or tendinitis. Adjust the resistance accordingly.

> ### SHOULDER PROTOCOLS
>
> The following exercises (Flexion, Abduction, Empty Can, and Internal and External Rotation) are standard in the rehabilitation of the shoulder. Each exercise isolates a specific muscle or muscle group that helps stabilize the shoulder joint. These exercises should initially be done without weight. Once the area is stronger, move to low weight (1 to 3 lbs.) or use light resistive surgical tubing. The exercises are shown with tubing, but weights (even canned goods weighing 1+ lbs.) can be used.

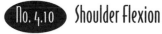 **No. 4.10** Shoulder Flexion

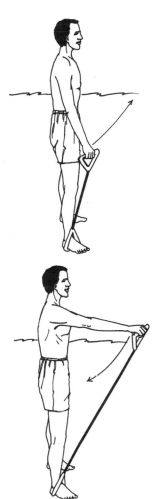

Equipment: Use the stretch cords or surgical tubing with this exercise.

Position: Spread the feet shoulder-width apart for support in above-the-waist to chest-high water.

Description: Slowly raise your arm directly in front of your body to shoulder height; you do not need to raise it any higher than this. Remember to keep the arm straight and the elbow locked. Control is the key; raise and lower the arm slowly. Repeat 10-20 times or to your tolerance.

Note: It is important not to compensate for shoulder weakness. Arching the back, leaning to the side, or jerking the arm quickly are forms of compensation.

Precautions: You will definitely feel this exercise! However, if pain persists or you have pain or loss of motion at this joint, see a doctor. If left unattended, it may develop into a "frozen shoulder."

No. 4.11 Shoulder Abduction

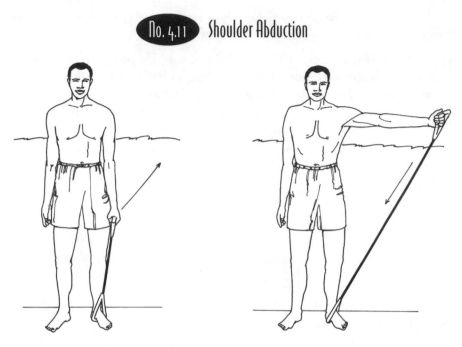

Equipment: Use the stretch cords or surgical tubing with this exercise.

Position: Stand in above-the-waist to chest-high water. Your arm is directly out to the side of your body with the elbow locked and the thumb pointing up.

Description: Raise the arm directly out and away from the body to a 90-degree angle (shoulder height). As you raise the straightened arm, the hand will be in a "thumbs up" position. Lower the arm slowly; remember, control is the key. Repeat 10-20 times, or to your tolerance. This exercise may be difficult. It is important to keep the elbow locked and the arm straight. Remember—thumbs up; this is critical to the exercise.

Note: It is important not to use the trunk of the body to compensate for shoulder weakness. Things like arching the back, leaning to the side, or jerking the arm up instead of keeping the up-and-down motion slow and controlled are forms of compensation.

Precautions: You will definitely feel this exercise! However, if pain persists or you have had pain or loss of motion at this joint, you need to see a doctor. Shoulders have minds of their own and if left unattended, it may develop into a "frozen shoulder." Take care of it now!

No. 4.12 Shoulder Empty Can

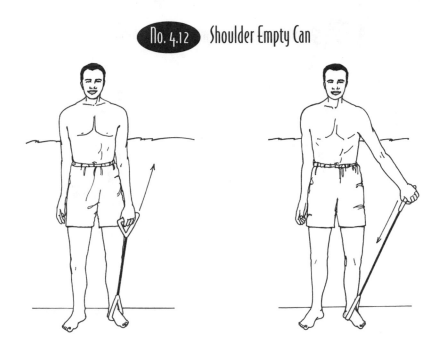

Equipment: Use the stretch cords or surgical tubing with this exercise.

Position: Position the arm at a 45-degree angle, or halfway between the front of the thigh and the outside of the thigh. The arm is rotated inward with the thumb against the thigh. The arm is straight and the elbow locked. You should be standing in above-the-waist to chest-high water.

Description: This exercise isolates the muscle in the back of the shoulder joint. Turn your arm so that you are leading with your little finger as you lift up and away at a 45-degree angle. If you are doing this correctly, you will feel it directly behind the shoulder joint. Lower the arm slowly and repeat. Remember, lock the elbow and keep the arm straight. You lead with the little finger as you raise the arm.

Note: It is important not to use the trunk of the body to compensate for shoulder weakness. Things like arching the back, leaning to the side, or jerking the arm up instead of keeping the up-and-down motion slow and controlled are forms of compensation.

Precautions: If pain persists or you have had pain or loss of motion at this joint, see a doctor. Shoulders have minds of their own and if left unattended, it may develop into a "frozen shoulder." Take care of it now!

No. 4.13 Internal and External Shoulder Rotation

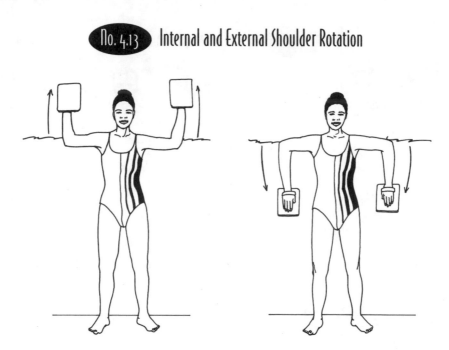

Equipment: Use hand paddles or webbed gloves if you want increased resistance with this exercise.

Position: Stand in chest-high water with your back flat against the wall. The arms are at shoulder level and the back and upper arms are flat against the pool wall.

Description: While keeping the elbow and upper arm against the pool wall, raise the forearm up toward the ear as high as possible. Now, press the forearm and hand into the water and push down until you touch the pool wall. Remember, the elbow and upper arm remain at shoulder level, pressed against the wall. Repeat, raising your forearm and hand up toward your ear. You should resemble a traffic cop with an arm in the *stop* position. Repeat 10-20 times on each arm, or to your tolerance. Hand paddles or webbed gloves add more resistance.

Note: It is important to keep the elbow and upper arm level with the shoulder as much as possible. This exercise works the rotator muscles of the shoulder, rotating the arm down or up toward the head.

Precautions: If you feel a sharp pain or pinch in front of the shoulder joint, lower the upper arm and elbow slightly so they are not at a 90-degree angle. However, remember to keep the elbow against the wall even if you have to lower it.

END OF SHOULDER EXERCISES

No. 4.14   Hip Extension With Cords (Pull-Backs)

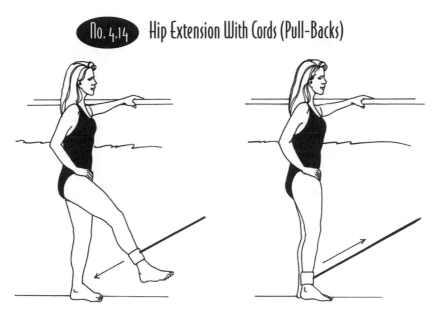

Equipment: Use the stretch cords or the surgical tubing with this exercise. You will need a strap to anchor the tubing to the leg.

Position: Hook your cord to a fixed and stable object, such as a handrail by the pool steps or a pool ladder in the shallow end of the pool. Secure the Velcro attachment around your ankle, positioning the buckle in front. Back away from the ladder/handrail slowly with that leg extended out in front of you. The cord should be taut with tension and the leg extended.

Description: Hold on to the side of the pool for support and slowly pull the leg down until it is even with the other leg. Both knees are locked when doing this exercise. Do not extend the leg behind the body, just bring it down even with the other leg. Release the leg slowly and repeat. Repeat 10-20 times, to your tolerance, then switch and do the other leg.

Note: For this exercise to be effective, the cord must have some tension in it when the leg is out in front of the body. Hold on to the side of the pool for support and maintain an upright posture! Check yourself to be sure you are not bending at the hips or waist. Otherwise, you may feel tension in your back.

Precautions: The exercise puts the hamstring (back of the thigh) on full stretch and works it against resistance. Start slowly because you are likely to experience some muscle soreness the first time or two you do this exercise.

No. 4.15 Hip Flexion With Cords (Pull-Forwards)

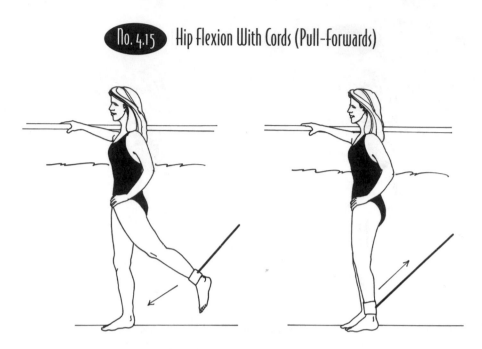

Equipment: Use the stretch cords or surgical tubing with this exercise. Use an ankle strap to hook onto the cord.

Position: This exercise is similar to the hip extension—only reversed. Again, attach your cord to a fixed and stable object such as a handrail or pool ladder in the shallow end.

Description: Secure the Velcro attachment around your ankle with the buckle positioned in back of the ankle. Extend the leg that is attached to the cord behind you. Slowly walk away from the ladder with your leg extended behind you until you feel tension in the cord. Keeping an upright posture (don't bend at the hips), pull the cord forward until the leg is even with the other, stabilizing leg. Again, keep both legs straight and knees locked. Release the leg up slowly and repeat 10-20 times, then switch the cord to the other leg.

Note: It is important to *keep the back straight* and maintain an upright posture. Otherwise, you make this exercise much harder than it is and create additional strain in the lower back area.

Precautions: Be sure your hips are squared and pointing straight ahead. Weakness in the muscles or trunk may allow the trunk to rotate and this affects the targeted muscle group. Do not raise the leg high behind you; this causes you to rotate the trunk.

No. 4.16 Hip Abduction With Cords (Pull-Outs)

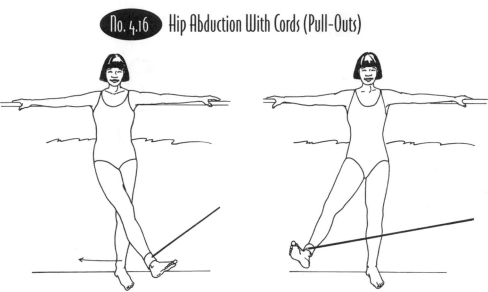

Equipment: Use the stretch cords or surgical tubing with some type of ankle attachment on this exercise.

Position: Attach your stretch cord to a secure object in the shallow end of the pool, with your back against the pool wall. Secure the Velcro attachment around your ankle with the buckle positioned on the inside. The right leg is stretched in front of and across the body. Step away from the handrail/ladder until you feel tension in the cord.

Description: With your back supported against the wall, pull across until the right leg is lined up with the right side of your body. Do not extend the leg away from the trunk of the body; it is not necessary to pull the cord that far. Return slowly to the original starting position and repeat 10-20 times. To switch to the left leg, turn and face the wall. Again, the velcro attachment is secured around the left ankle and the buckle positioned on the inside of the ankle. Pull across the body until the left leg lines up with the left side of your body. Relax the leg as it returns to the original starting position and repeat 10-20 times, according to your tolerance.

Note: Lean against the pool wall when you do the right leg, then face the wall when you do the left leg. The exercise works each leg, and each side of the trunk.

Precautions: This exercise is very difficult. Remember to keep the legs straight and knees locked. If this exercise causes any pain or discomfort, review the instructions to make sure you are following proper positioning. Discontinue if the exercise remains painful.

Hip Adduction With Cords (Pull-Ins)

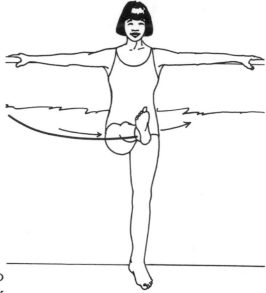

Equipment: Use the stretch cords or tubing with some type of ankle attachment.

Position: Attach stretch cord to a handrail or pool ladder in the shallow end of the pool. Lean your back against the pool wall.

Description: Secure the Velcro attachment around the left ankle with the buckle positioned on the outside of the ankle. Your left leg is straight and extended out to the side of the body. Back away from the handrail/pool ladder with the left leg extended out until you feel tension in the cord. Keep your body upright against the pool wall and your leg out straight. Pull in toward the body until the leg lines up with the mid-line of the body (navel, nose, etc.). Relax your left leg slowly away from your body and repeat 10-20 times, to your tolerance. To switch to the right leg, turn and face the pool wall. Secure the velcro attachment to your right ankle with the buckle positioned on the outside of the ankle. Your right leg is straight and extended away from your body. Adjust your position so that there is tension in the stretch cord. Pull the right leg in slowly to mid-line (nose, navel) and then release out to the original starting position. Repeat 10-20 times, to your tolerance. Remember, do not bend at the hips or turn the body.

Note: You are against the wall when you do the left leg and facing the wall when you do the right leg. It may seem confusing, but after a couple of times, this exercise will make sense and all confusion should end.

Precautions: Use the pool wall for support when you do this exercise; it helps protect the back. Again, if you experience any kind of pain or discomfort, discontinue the exercise.

No. 4.18 Back Extension With Cords (Stick-Ups)

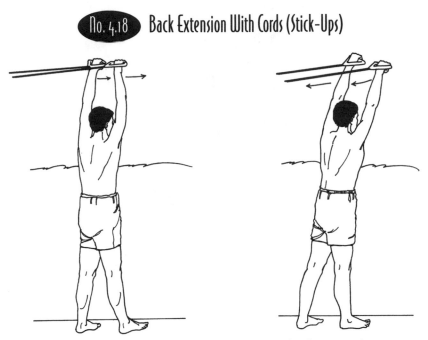

Equipment: Use the stretch cords or surgical tubing in this exercise. Preferably, use a stretch cord that has handles.

Position: Secure the cords to a fixed and stable object, such as a pool ladder or handrail in the shallow end of the pool. Step forward, away from the cords, with your back turned away and the cords behind you. Feet are shoulder-width apart and pointing straight ahead.

Description: Place the cord handles together and grasp in both hands. Extend the arms up to a point about 4-6 inches behind your head. This position will arch your back and open up the chest area to stretch. Lean slightly forward for leverage. With elbows locked, pull the cords forward about 4-6 inches so you can see your arms slightly in front of your head if you look up. This is a small controlled movement. Slowly release the cords back behind your head with elbows locked and repeat 10-20 times, according to your tolerance.

Note: It is very important that this exercise be done with the elbows locked. Otherwise, a different muscle group is used and that totally changes the exercise. Also, use a wider base of support for additional leverage.

Precautions: This exercise puts the back into extension. If you cannot do it in a slow, controlled manner, come back to it after your back is stronger. The exercise really targets all the trunk muscles, especially the abdominals.

No. 4.19   Heel Walks

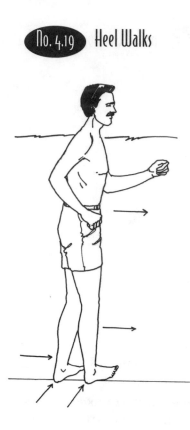

Position: Stand in water about chest high.

Description: Walk on the heels only across the pool. Turn around and return while continuing to walk on your heels. The knees are locked and the legs are stiff. You do not walk backward on your heels, only forward.

Note: This exercise works the muscle that runs parallel to the shin or tibia. This is a good exercise for those people who repeatedly get "shin splints," or Achilles tendinitis.

Precautions: None, really. Start slowly if you are working to resolve "shin splints." This muscle can be easily overloaded and inflamed. Pace yourself and incorporate this exercise into your routine gradually.

No. 4.20 Carioca

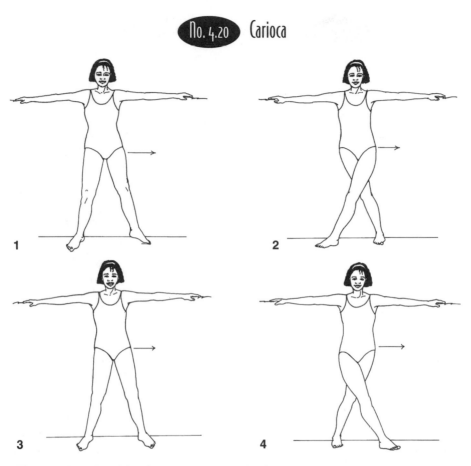

1

2

3

4

Position: Stand sideways in chest-high water.

Description: Take a normal step sideways with the left leg. The legs remain as straight as possible. Now cross the right leg behind the left; step sideways again with the left leg. This time, cross the right leg in front. Continue alternating across the pool, step, step-behind, step, step-front. When you get to the other side of the pool, start back across, this time leading with the right leg. Remember, step, step-behind, step, step-front. Repeat 4-5 times over and back across the pool, or for about 5-10 minutes.

Note: Remember to keep your shoulders squared. The pelvis will rotate around the stationary trunk. Do not turn the upper body. This allows more stretch through the back and hips and is an excellent exercise for balance problems.

Precautions: None. This may be difficult if your back or hips are inflexible. Perseverance pays off; just go at your own pace.

No. 4.21 Lateral Trunk Flexion (Hula Dancer)

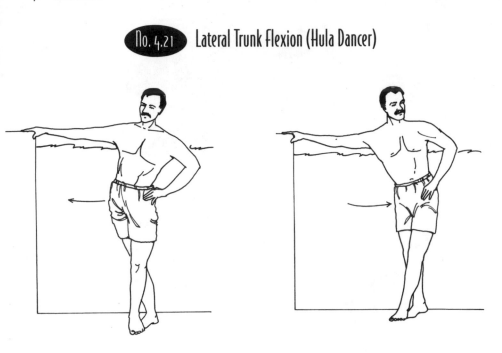

Position: Stand sideways along the pool wall in above-the-waist to chest-high water. The right leg is closest to the wall and is slightly behind the left leg.

Description: While leaning on the right arm or elbow, drop the hips toward the wall as far as you comfortably can (well, reasonably comfortably—there is no such thing as comfortably). Heels and feet remain flat on the pool floor. Hold for 5-10 seconds, then push back to the original starting position. Repeat about 10 times and hold each stretch 10-15 seconds. Now switch and do the other side.

Note: By placing the leg closest to the pool wall slightly behind the other, you enable the body to get a full stretch on that area from the hip to the knee. This exercise is excellent for people experiencing pain along the outside (lateral) surface of the hip and upper thigh and knee. Just make believe you are a hula dancer and shift those hips!

Precautions: Ease into the stretch slowly. If you have a tight hip or painful knee, you will definitely feel a pull. That is why you need to ease into the stretch by shifting your hips over toward the wall. Feet stay as flat as possible.

No. 4.22 Behind the Back Push-Downs

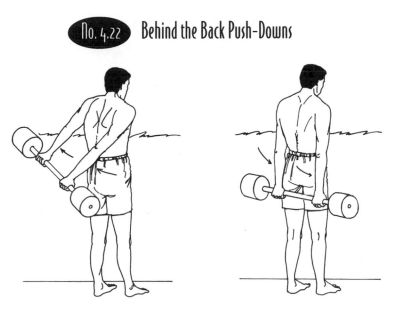

Equipment: Use a large floating barbell. You can substitute hand barbells or a small plastic ball, too.

Position: Stand in water waist high to above the waist. The floating barbell is behind you with your hands grasping the float, palms down. Your elbows are locked, your arms are straight, and your posture is upright.

Description: With the body in an upright position, press the barbell down toward your hips, keeping your arms straight. Keep the back straight. Relax the barbell up and repeat 10-20 times. Hold behind you for 1-2 minutes (if possible!) for a static stretch of the upper back, chest, and shoulders, or you can repeat up to 20 repetitions for something a little easier.

Note: This exercise is excellent, and *difficult*, for individuals with rounded shoulders. That's what your mother called "slumping." Mom knew what she was talking about! Poor posture develops into problems over time. Keep your back straight in this exercise. If you cannot straighten up, move to shallower water until you can get your arms completely straight, elbows locked, and posture upright!

Precautions: This may be too aggressive for shoulder patients. If you continue to have discomfort after moving to shallower water, wait awhile before starting this exercise. After your back loosens up, you will be able to do this. Also, if this causes discomfort in the elbows, move to shallow water or discontinue.

No. 4.23   Hop Scotch

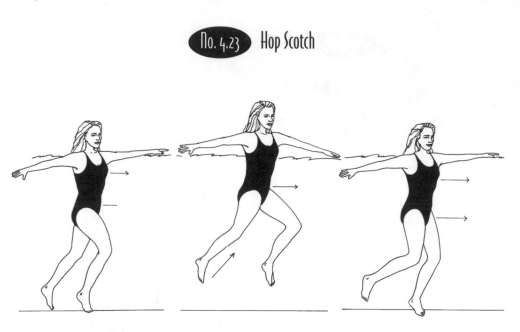

Position: Stand in water above the waist to chest high.

Description: Hop onto one leg, push upward, come back to both feet, then hop onto the other leg. Continue all the way across the pool and back. Repeat several times. Use the whole foot—no tip-toes!

Note: This exercise is excellent for strengthening a weak ankle, knee, or hip. It allows for short rest breaks as you isolate the weak joint.

Precautions: Do not start off with this exercise. Build up your lower extremity strength first through squats, single leg squats, and lunges, then move to this exercise. This is a good aerobic exercise if you do not rest much (15-30 seconds maximum) in between trips across the pool.

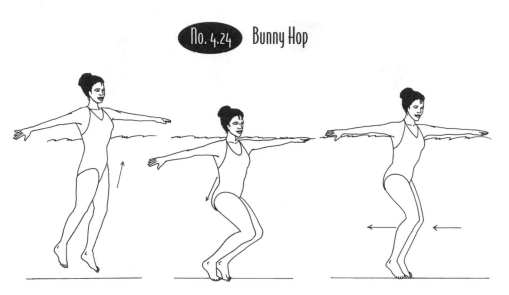

No. 4.24 Bunny Hop

Position: Stand in water above the waist to chest high.

Description: Starting with the feet together, bend the knees, push up and jump forward, landing on both feet. Repeat across the pool. Now, return to your original starting position by jumping backward across the pool. This works the hips and entire leg.

Note: This will also be a bit of an aerobic exercise. Proceed at your own pace. The shorter the rest break, the more aerobic the workout. Use your arms as much as you like. If you want the exercise to be more challenging, use your legs only. Put your arms behind your back or neck.

Precautions: This is an intermediate exercise. Build up your ankles, knees, hips, and back by starting out with squats and lunges. Work up to this exercise after you have established a foundation of strength.

No. 4.25 Lateral Step-Ups

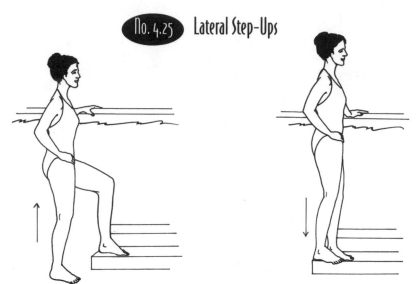

Equipment: Use a large brick, block, or step stool if your pool does not have steps.

Position: Go to the pool steps in the shallow end. Place involved or injured leg up on the step, with the knee flexed. The other leg is fully extended with the foot flat and pointing straight ahead.

Description: Straighten the involved knee (the one on the step) to an upright position. This will raise the strong leg up to the step level. Do not place the strong leg on the step. Slowly, lower the strong leg down until the foot is flat on the ground. If at all possible, do not hold onto anything for support; control the movement through the strength of the involved leg (the one on the step). If you must hold on, use one hand only. Repeat 10-20 times, to your tolerance. You may switch and do the uninvolved or stronger leg if you would like—it is optional on this exercise.

Note: This exercise is good for weak knees, hips, or ankles. The key to this exercise is controlling the movement and rate of speed. If you are unable to control the movement of lowering the foot down flat on the pool floor, then lower it down until your tip-toes touch, then repeat. Your knee, hip, or ankle may not be strong enough to control the movement through the full range.

Precautions: This is a very challenging exercise. If you have pain under or below the kneecap (patella), discontinue. This may be aggravating an acutely inflamed condition. This exercise is good for people who have problems with stairs. Also, start with smaller steps if possible in the beginning. Bend the knee and hip to a 45-degree angle only. Do not do a deep-knee bend with this exercise.

No. 4.26 One-Legged Stork

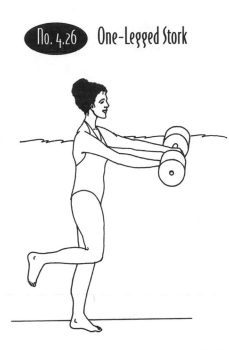

Equipment: You can use a large floating barbell, kickboard, or hand barbells with this exercise if you need additional support for balance.

Position: This depends on your balance, essentially. Start in waist-high to above-the-waist water. Use one to two floating barbells to assist you in keeping your balance. Feet are flat and pointing straight ahead.

Description: Lift one leg off the pool floor and bend it. The other leg is completely straight and is now bearing all your weight. Hold 10, 15, 20, 45, or 60 seconds and release down. Hold the leg up and balance as long as you can before resting. The number of seconds you hold this position depends on you and your balance. Now switch and balance on the other leg the same number of seconds, if possible. Alternate legs, doing a total of 5-7 balances on each side. Keep the foot firmly planted during this exercise—no little hops to regain your balance.

Note: This is an excellent exercise for strengthening the ankle, knee, or hip. It is also good for improving balance. The deeper the water on this exercise, the less control you have. If you have difficulty keeping your balance, move to shallower water and use the barbells to help you. You want to work toward doing this exercise without assistance. No fair holding onto the wall!

Precautions: If you have an acutely tender ankle, knee, or hip, you might wait to do this exercise until the area/joint is not so tender.

No. 4.27 Lunges

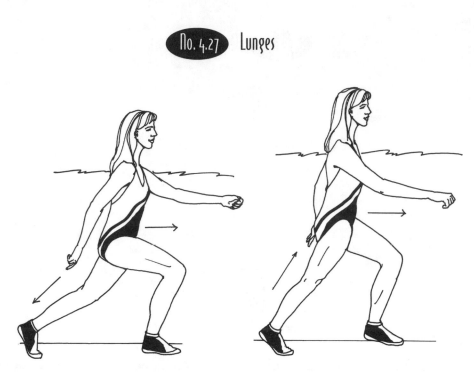

Equipment: Use hand barbells or large floating barbells if you need additional support and balance.

Position: Move to the shallow end of the pool, about 3-4 feet deep.

Description: Take a normal step forward and slowly bend the front leg down, as if going down on one knee. The back knee does not touch the bottom of the pool. Then, slowly straighten the front leg to a standing position and bring the back leg forward and start stepping out again. Slowly drop down, but do not touch the knee to the floor of the pool. Extend the front leg up into a standing position and repeat. Alternate legs across the shallow end of the pool 2-3 times (over and back), to your tolerance.

Note: There should be no stopping after coming into a standing position. This exercise requires control, balance, and hip and lower extremity strength. You can stop between steps if necessary, or use some equipment to help you with balance.

Precautions: This exercise may be hard on knee or hip patients who go into a deep-knee bend (90-degree angle). Move to slightly deeper water (4 feet) and drop down to about a 45-degree angle only (slightly bent knee). This will be easier on the knees and hips. Remember, heels stay flat on the pool floor—do not step in a tip-toe fashion.

No. 4.28   Sitting Abdominal and Hip Crunches

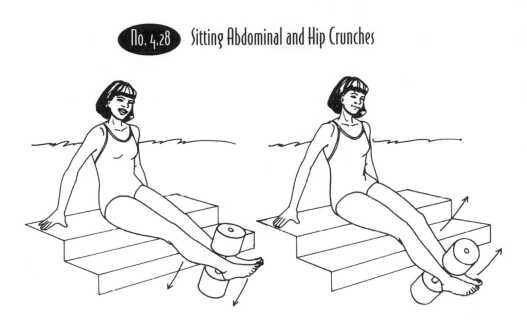

Equipment: Use a pull-buoy or one hand barbell with this exercise.

Position: Sit on the edge of the lower steps in the pool's shallow end. Place the pull-buoy between your ankles. Your knees are locked and the legs straight. Place your arms behind you and lean slightly forward to counteract the float.

Description: Leaning slightly forward with your arms behind you for support, push the float down to the bottom of the pool—remember, your knees are locked and your legs are straight. Slowly let the float up—knees are locked! Do not let the float go all the way to the surface— keep it underwater. Repeat 10-20 times, to your tolerance.

Note: Do this exercise *slowly* or the float will throw you off balance! Use your arms behind you to counteract the float (pull-buoy).

Precautions: You will feel this in your lower abdominals and lower back. If lower back pain increases, it will be best to come back to this exercise after you have gotten stronger. Do not do this exercise if it causes sharp leg pain!

No. 4.29 Windmills

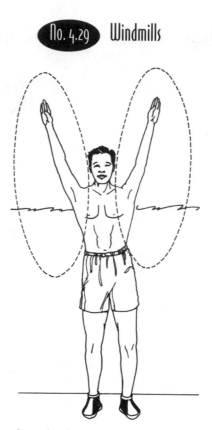

Position: Stand in chest-high water with your feet shoulder-width apart and pointing straight ahead. Arms are straight with the elbows locked.

Description: Raise your arms up simultaneously out of the water and make a full reaching sweep through the air and back down into the water, tracing a large circle from the hips, above the head, and down. Repeat 10-20 times, to your tolerance (you'll work on this one, believe me!). Now reverse arms and trace large circles from the hip to overhead, in a counter-clockwise direction. A wide base of support really helps here.

Note: This exercise is good but difficult for a lot of people, especially for those with shoulder or neck problems. Moving to shallower water should make it easier. If the exercise is still difficult, raise the arms to shoulder level only and make large circles clockwise and counter-clockwise below the water's surface. Avoid overhead motions.

Precautions: If this exercise causes increased neck or shoulder pain, discontinue completely.

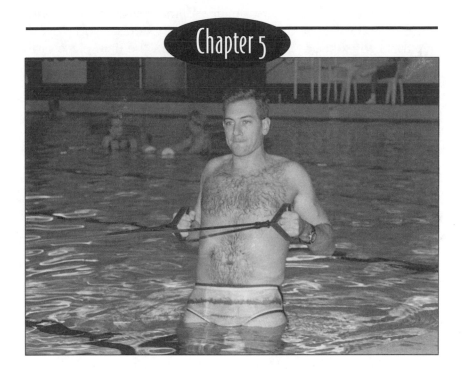

Chapter 5

Advanced Exercises

The exercises in the advanced portion of the program require flexibility, strength, and endurance. By the time you have progressed to this level, you should have developed the necessary tools to successfully and safely perform these exercises.

There are a few exercises that require equipment, but the majority of the advanced program focuses on trunk strength and stability or control. Many of the exercises require you to balance and sustain a certain position while performing another task or movement simultaneously.

Stabilization of the trunk, or control, requires the back extensors and abdominal musculature to work concurrently. The harmony of the muscles working together helps stabilize the spine and weaker areas against possible reinjury. You must learn how to move safely with an injured back and how to move to prevent a back injury. Without strength and control of the trunk, you will have difficulty doing these exercises correctly.

The advanced exercises in chapter 5 represent the final piece of the puzzle for a good and safe fitness or rehabilitative program.

The exercises and the pages on which they appear follow.

No. 5.1 Warm-Up Laps

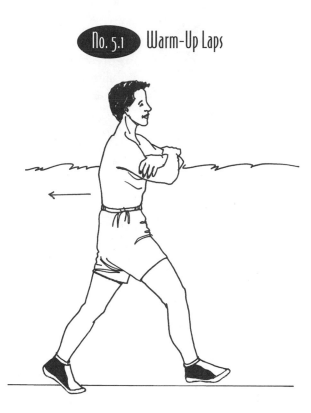

Position: Stand in chest-high water.

Description: Cross your arms over your chest. Walk across the pool. When you reach the other side, walk backward across the water to your starting point. When walking backward, keep the knees locked and the legs stiff.

Note: You will feel this exercise more when walking backward. Try taking smaller steps, but do continue with the stiff-legged gait.

Precautions: Your back will go into extension when walking backward. If you feel some discomfort, take smaller steps. If discomfort persists, abandon the stiff-legged gait and just walk backward with bent knees.

Advanced Note: By taking the arms out of this exercise, you will further recruit the trunk and legs, which will provide the power to move against the resistance of the water. Tighten the abdominals to help strengthen the stability of the trunk as you move through the water.

No. 5.2 Carioca

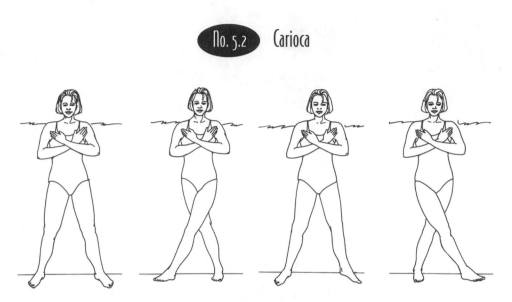

Position: Stand sideways in chest-high water with your arms folded across the chest.

Description: Take a normal step sideways with the left leg. The legs remain as straight as possible. Now cross the right leg behind the back; step sideways again with the left leg. This time, cross the right leg in front of the body. Continue alternating across the pool, step, step-behind, step, step-front. When you get to the other side of the pool, start back across, this time leading with the left leg. Remember, step, step-behind, step, step-front. Repeat 4-5 times over and back across the pool, or work about 5-10 minutes.

Note: Remember to keep your shoulders squared. The pelvis will rotate around the stationary trunk. Do not rotate the shoulders—the upper body is still! This allows more stretch through the back and hips. This exercise is excellent for balance problems.

Precautions: None. This may be difficult if your back or hips are inflexible. Perseverance pays off; just go at your own pace.

Advanced Note: Again, the arms have been taken out of this exercise. Balance and momentum come from the strength and stability of the trunk. The power to move through the water comes from the legs, hips, and lower back.

No. 5.3 Lunges

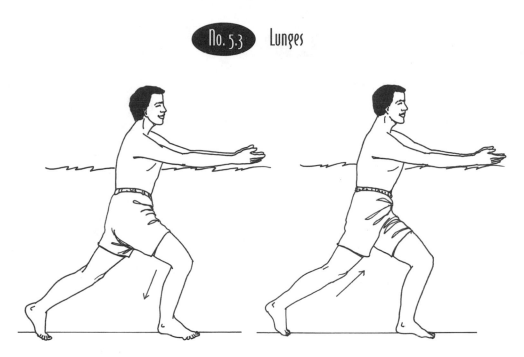

Position: Move to shallow water, about 3-4 ft. deep. Hold arms straight in front of you at shoulder level. The elbows are locked and fingers laced together.

Description: Take a normal step forward and slowly bend the front knee. The back knee does not touch the bottom of the pool. Then, slowly extend the front leg to a standing position and bring the back leg forward and start stepping out again. Slowly drop down, but do not touch the knee to the floor of the pool. Extend your front leg up into a standing position and repeat. Alternate legs across the shallow end of the pool 2-3 times (over and back), to your tolerance.

Note: There should be no stopping after coming into an upright position. This exercise requires control, balance, and hip and lower extremity strength. If you cannot do this exercise without stopping between steps, try to work up to that level.

Precautions: Move to slightly deeper water if this bothers your hips or knees.

Advanced Note: Recognize a pattern, here? Once again, the arms are out of this exercise to fully recruit the strength and stability of the trunk, and the power of the legs. Tighten the abdominals to further stabilize the trunk and pelvis.

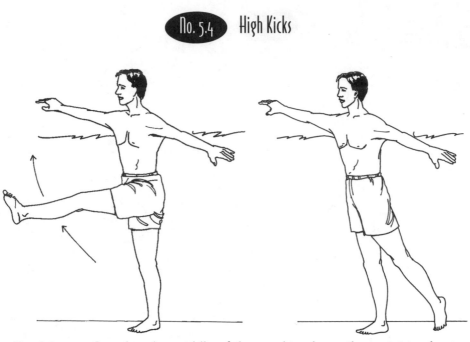

No. 5.4   High Kicks

Position: Stand in the middle of the pool in above-the-waist to chest-high water.

Description: Pull the foot up tight (as opposed to pointing it), and lift the leg up as high as it can comfortably go. The knee is locked and the opposite leg is straight with the heel down. The back should remain straight—no leaning forward or backward when kicking. After kicking forward, push the leg backward in one continuous motion. It is not necessary to kick back far. Again, the back stays straight—keep an upright posture. Continue with 20-30 repetitions on the same leg, then switch to the other leg.

Note: If you are unable to raise the leg very high due to hamstring tightness, that's okay. It is more important that you maintain an upright position. This exercise strengthens the quadriceps (front of the thigh), hamstrings (back of the thigh), hips, and entire trunk.

Precautions: Do not extend your leg very far behind you. It is not necessary and can be uncomfortable. About 12 inches is adequate.

Advanced Note: Remember—tighten your abdominals, low back, and buttocks to help stabilize the trunk and provide a solid base from which to move. Use your arms as needed to help you with your balance.

No. 5.5 Hip In and Outs

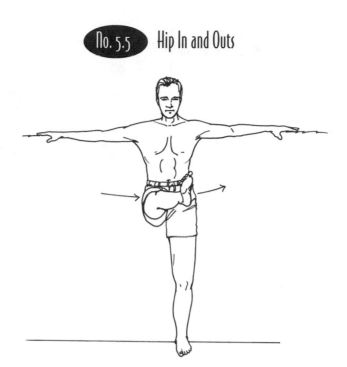

Position: Stand in the middle of the pool in above-the-waist to chest-high water.

Description: Raise the leg as high as is comfortably possible. Pull the foot back—do not point the toe. Swing the leg out away from the body, then swing back in one continuous motion. Continue with 20-30 repetitions on the same leg, then switch to the other leg. To maintain an erect posture, swing your arms in the opposite motion of the leg. For example, if kicking the leg out to the right, move the arms to the left to counteract that motion. It's like an old-fashioned "twist."

Note: It is not necessary to swing your leg very far away from your body. It is more important to swing it across your whole body to get a full stretch on the hip and lower back. This exercise is for the inner and outer thigh and hips. We can all use this exercise!

Precautions: This exercise may be uncomfortable for acute lower back patients. Nor should you do this exercise if you have had a total hip replacement. Proceed with caution if you have back problems. Do not do this if you have had recent back surgery or a recent herniated disc.

Advanced Note: Remember—tighten the abdominals, low back, and buttocks to help stabilize the trunk and provide a solid base from which to move.

No. 5.6   Shoulder Press-Downs

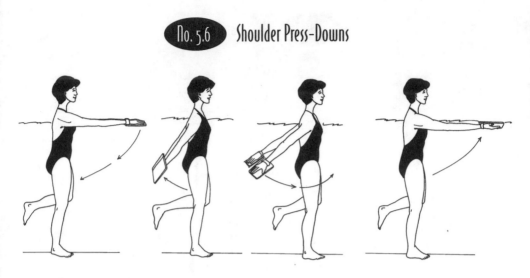

Equipment: You can use hand paddles with this exercise to make it harder.

Position: Stand on one leg in water above the waist to chest high and lock the knee. Hold the arms out in front of the body with the elbow locked and palms facing down.

Description: Press your arms and hands down toward the hips, keeping the arms close to the sides. When the hands and arms are parallel to the hips, flip the hands over and, keeping the elbows locked, push the arms up to the surface of the water. Repeat 20-30 times, to your tolerance. Keep the foot of the leg you are standing on planted—no little bounces to help keep your balance.

Note: If you tend to lose your balance on this exercise, move in a bit to shallower water. If you need the exercise to be more challenging, use large hand paddles or move into deeper water.

Precautions: This is all about balance and learning to adjust when your center of gravity changes. Shorten the arm strokes here and move to shallower water to compensate for the leg that was taken away!

Advanced Note: Remember, tighten your abdominals, low back, and buttocks to help stabilize the trunk and provide a solid base from which to move.

No. 5.7   Abdominal Press-Downs

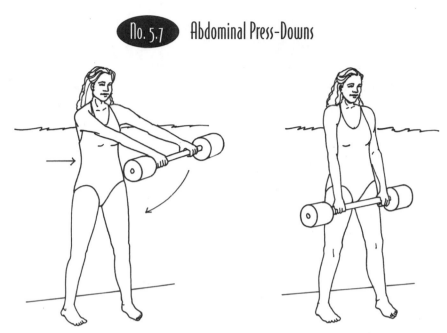

Equipment: You can use a large floating barbell or plastic ball with this exercise.

Position: Stand in the middle of the pool in above-the-waist to chest-high water. Spread the feet shoulder-width apart. The floating barbell is held at arm's length from the body, with the elbows locked.

Description: Push the float under the water and down to the hips, if possible. Slowly, allow the float to rise and repeat the exercise, *keeping the elbows locked*, 10-20 times, to your tolerance. You will feel this one immediately in the abdominals. Persevere, it gets easier.

Note: This is an excellent abdominal and trunk-strengthening exercise. It helps those flabby upper arms as well. If you cannot get the float underwater, move to shallower water. To make the exercise more difficult, move out deeper and/or put your feet together.

Precautions: Do not cheat on this exercise by leaning forward and using your body weight for leverage. This exercise uses both the abdominals and back extensors simultaneously. Move to shallower water or discontinue if this increases your lower back discomfort.

Advanced Note: Remember to tighten your abdominals, low back, and buttocks to help stabilize the trunk and provide a solid base from which to move. Be sure you don't "power" the float under by leaning forward and using your body weight for leverage. A strong, anchored trunk and upper back will enable you to perform this exercise.

Chest Flys Modified

Equipment: Use hand paddles with this exercise to make it more difficult.

Position: Stand on one leg in above-the-waist to chest-high water, with the foot pointing straight ahead. Hand paddles should be secured on each hand with the palms facing outward and the elbows locked.

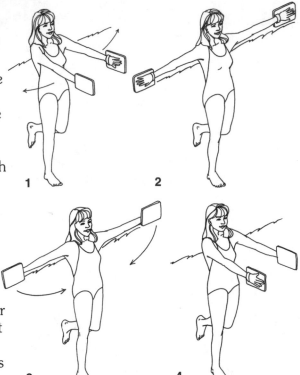

Description: Slowly push the arms back and away from you with the paddles just under the surface of the water. After your arms are directly out to your sides, turn the paddles over so the palms are coming in together as you push the water forward. Repeat, turning the palms over so they are facing away from each other and push straight arms back and away. Repeat 20-30 times.

Note: Tighten the lower back and buttocks and lean into the exercise at the hips when you are pushing the hands forward and together. Shorten the strokes you make with the paddles to compensate for the very narrow base of support—one leg!

Precautions: If you are having trouble keeping your balance, move to shallower water for better leverage.

Advanced Note: Remember to tighten your abdominals, low back, and buttocks to help stabilize the trunk and provide a solid base from which to move.

Squats

Position: Stand in the middle of the pool in 3-4 ft. of water. Your feet should be pointing straight ahead, not rotated and pointing outward. Stand with the feet 4-6 in. apart.

Description: Squat down as far as you can comfortably go, while keeping the *heels down*. If you reach a point where your heels begin to pull up off the pool floor, do not go any further; this will be your maximum point of flexion. To make this exercise harder, hold your arms straight out in front of you with the elbows locked and fingers laced together. Now you must rely on the strength of your legs and trunk to help you maintain your balance while performing the exercise. Squat down as far as you can comfortably go while keeping the heels down.

Note: This exercise is to be done slowly. If you do it quickly, you use momentum rather than strength and it isn't as effective overall. In fact, that's cheating.

Precautions: This exercise may be bothersome for anyone with arthritic knees or patellar (kneecap) problems. Those individuals should move to slightly deeper (above-the-waist) water and squat to a 45-degree angle only versus a deep-knee bend. Do not do this exercise if it is too painful.

Advanced Note: Remember to tighten your abdominals, low back, and buttocks to help stabilize the trunk and provide a solid base from which to move.

Squats With Ball: To make this exercise harder, hold a ball straight out in front of you. As you squat down, raise the ball up over your head. As you stand up, lower the ball to waist level. Now you must rely on the strength of your legs and trunk to help you maintain your balance.

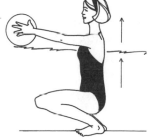

No. 5.10   Cheerleading Squats

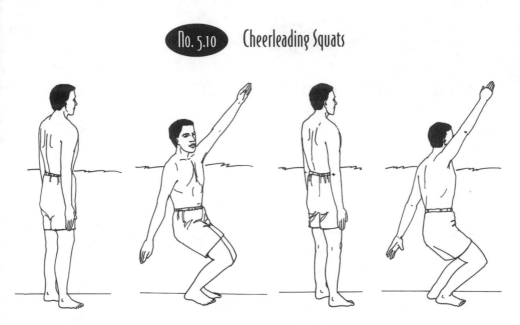

Position: Stand in the middle of the pool in 3-4 ft. of water. Feet are pointing straight ahead, not rotated or pointing outward. Stand with the feet 4-6 in. apart.

Description: Squat down as far as you can comfortably go, keeping the heels down. To make this exercise even harder, as you squat and rise, swing your arms up and down. You must use the trunk and legs for balance and control.

Note: If you need to make this exercise even *harder*, speed up your arm swings when squatting. The faster the motion, the more control and trunk strength you will need to complete this exercise.

Precautions: This exercise may be bothersome for individuals with arthritic knees or patellar (kneecap) problems. Do not do this exercise if it is too painful.

Advanced Note: Remember to tighten your abdominals, low back, and buttocks to help stabilize the trunk and provide a solid base from which to move.

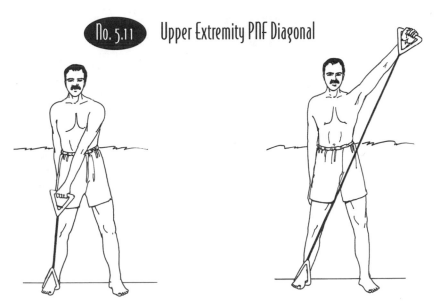

No. 5.11 Upper Extremity PNF Diagonal

Equipment: Use stretch cord or surgical tubing with this exercise.

Position: Stand in water above the waist to chest high. Feet are shoulder-width apart. The hips are slightly tucked under, abdominals tightened, and knees slightly bent. Place the rubber tubing under one foot and grasp the other end with the opposite hand. For example, if the cord is anchored under the left foot, the right arm is across the body with the hand in front of the left hip.

Description: The motion of this exercise is from low to high. Pull the tether cord up and across the body, and end with the arm fully extended above the right shoulder at an angle. Repeat 5-10 times, then switch to the left arm. Remember, always work both sides of the body. Now, the cord is across the body with the hand in front of the right hip. Go from low to high and keep the arm as straight as possible. Lower the arm and repeat 5-10 times.

Note: This exercise works the extensors and rotators of the trunk, the abdominals, and the upper back. If you cannot lift your arm above your head, lift it to shoulder level or slightly above, hold for 5 seconds, and lower. By working in a diagonal pattern, you strengthen both the front and back of the trunk.

Precautions: If you cannot do this exercise in a controlled manner, move to shallower water. If you still have difficulty, hold off on this exercise. The trunk remains straight with the main movement at the arm and upper back. If you do this exercise without good control you will place the back in a vulnerable position.

No. 5.12   Frontal Diagonal Pulls

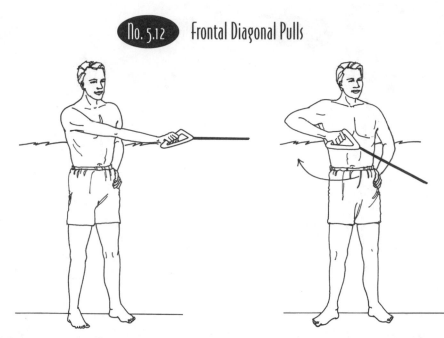

Equipment: Use stretch cord or surgical tubing with this exercise.

Position: Stand in waist-high water. Anchor the tether cord or rubber tubing to the pool railing or ladder. One arm is outstretched in front of the body diagonally, grasping the cord. Feet are shoulder-width apart, with the hips slightly tucked under. Back muscles and abdominals are tightened to help stabilize the trunk and hips.

Description: Pull the cord across the body in a diagonal pattern until the elbow is bent and slightly behind the trunk. Relax slowly back into the outstretched arm position, moving back across the body in a diagonal pattern. Feet remain firmly planted. There will be a rotation of the trunk and hips as the arm comes across and back. Repeat up to 20 times, then switch to the other arm. Be sure to work both sides of the body.

Note: This exercise works the rotator muscles of the trunk. Remember, the trunk is straight and tall with this exercise; it should be a nice controlled and flowing motion.

Precautions: If you cannot maintain an erect posture or are slightly bent at your knees or hips, do not do this exercise. If you are arching your back or if the motion is not smooth and controlled, do not do this exercise. These postures indicate some trunk weakness or lingering inflexibility. Do not do this exercise unless you can control the motion—to do otherwise places the back in a vulnerable position. Be smart!

No. 5.13   "X" Marks the Spot

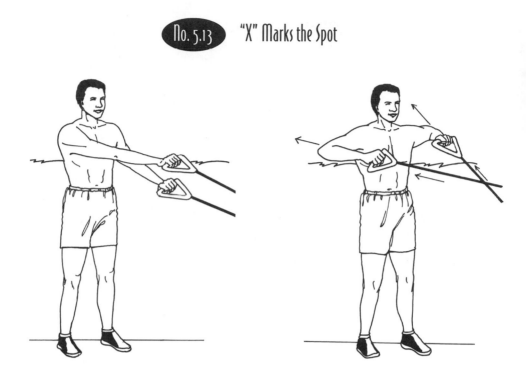

Equipment: Use stretch cords or surgical tubing with this exercise.

Position: Secure the cords to a fixed and stable object, such as a hand-rail or pool ladder in the shallow end of the pool. Slowly back away with your arms out straight while gripping the cord handles. Continue until the cords are taut. The feet are pointing straight ahead with the legs shoulder-width apart for leverage.

Description: Your arms are outstretched and crossed at the wrist, making an "X." With the arms outstretched and cords taut, slowly pull the cords back to the sides of the body at chest level. Release slowly to starting position and do 10-20 repetitions, or to your tolerance. You are working diagonally across the trunk.

Note: You will start with the palms down and end with the hands at chest level. If you start with the right hand on top, switch after 10-15 repetitions, and reposition so the left hand is on top.

Precautions: Be sure and get a wide base to give yourself some lever-age. Do this exercise in a slow, controlled movement.

Advanced Note: Remember to tighten your abdominals, low back, and buttocks to help stabilize the trunk and provide a solid base from which to move.

No. 5.14   Biceps Curl (Popeye)

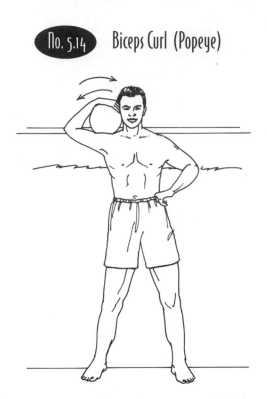

Equipment: Use a medium-sized plastic ball with this exercise.

Position: Stand against the pool wall in above-the-waist water to support the back and maintain correct overall posture.

Description: Place a medium-sized plastic ball over the biceps with the arm cradling the ball within the bend of the elbow and shoulder as illustrated. Press the wrist down into the ball, hold for 2-3 seconds, and release. Repeat the action up to 20 repetitions, then switch arms. Repeat with the other arm, holding the muscle contraction briefly, then relaxing. This is a pumping action.

Note: If you are working on your upper back, shoulder, and arm endurance, this is a good exercise. Do a rapid succession of repetitions on both sides. Be sure to hold the arm at a 90-degree angle at the side of the body.

Precautions: This is more of an aerobic exercise. Do not do this particular biceps exercise if you have problems with neck pain, or restrictions or pain with shoulder range of motion.

No. 5.15   Can-Can Dance

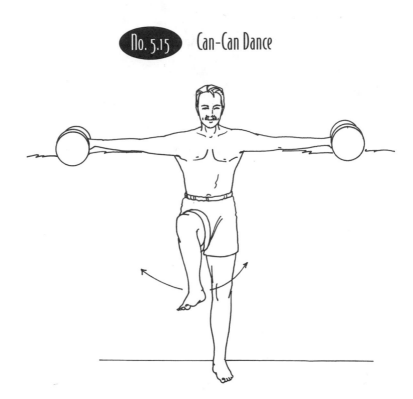

Equipment: Use two large floating barbells or your hand barbells to assist with balance.

Position: Stand in chest-high water and hold a barbell float directly out to each side.

Description: Raise one leg to a 90-degree angle of hip flexion. While keeping the hip and knee flexed to 90 degrees, turn the lower leg and ankle in, then out. Repeat 20 times then switch legs.

Note: By standing in the middle of the pool on one leg, you get two exercises in one. Not only are you dynamically exercising the hips, you are also strengthening the trunk by sustaining a fixed posture. You must use the abdominals and back extensors to stabilize and anchor the trunk while you balance on one leg to perform the dynamic movement.

Precautions: Do not do this exercise if you have had hip replacement surgery.

Advanced Note: Remember to tighten the abdominals, low back, and buttocks to help stabilize the trunk and provide a solid base from which to move.

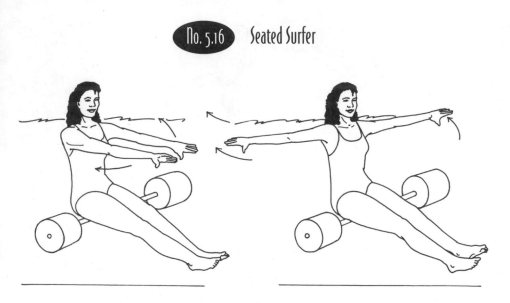

No. 5.16   Seated Surfer

Equipment: If possible, use a large floating barbell with this exercise.

Position: Get in about 4 ft. of water and place the barbell float under your buttocks so you are sitting on it like a chair. Raise your calves straight out in front of you, as if you were sitting on the floor.

Description: Position the arms straight in front of the body at shoulder height. Your position looks like a "C," balancing on top of the barbell. Face the palms away from each other with the thumbs pointing down toward the pool floor. Push the arms back and away to propel yourself across the water. Try to keep the legs out in front of you with knees locked. Proceed across the pool until you reach the other side. Now, the palms will be coming in toward the middle of the body with the thumbs up. You are now pulling your arms in front of the body and propelling yourself backward across the pool. Remember, keep the legs straight out in front of you as much as possible.

Note: If you have trouble balancing, you can bend your knees slightly for leverage. Be sure you can balance on the barbell first, then add the arms to the exercise.

Precautions: None. This exercise requires excellent trunk stability and lots of upper body strength.

Advanced Note: Remember to tighten the abdominals, low back, and buttocks to help stabilize the trunk and provide a solid base from which to move.

No. 5.17   Lower Extremity Squares

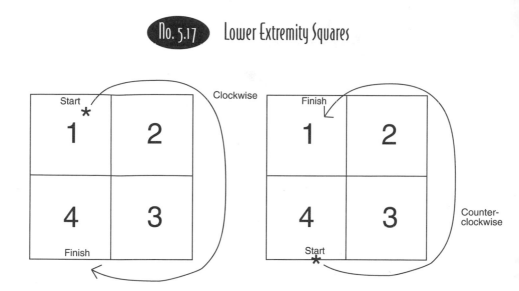

Position: Stand in waist-high water, away from the wall. Balance on the injured lower extremity, with the uninvolved leg bent behind you—as if you are playing hop scotch.

Description: Imagine four squares on the pool bottom, as illustrated. Jump clockwise, from square 1, to 2, to 3, to 4. Now, without stopping, reverse and jump counter-clockwise from square 4, to 3, to 2, and finish on square 1. Repeat, jumping from square 1 to 4, then reverse, going from square 4 to 1. Repeat 5 to 10 times without stopping. Rest and repeat a second set of 5 to 10 repetitions. Repeat the drill on the other leg.

Note: This is an aggressive exercise and should not be done as part of the beginner series. This is for intermediate to advanced levels and cross trainers. Do not do this exercise if you are having swelling in the joint on an ongoing basis. You can use this exercise for strengthening the ankles, knees, or hips; it works all these joints. To increase the difficulty and amount of weightbearing on the joint(s), move to shallower water.

Precautions: This is a higher-level exercise and should not be done until significant strength has been developed in the joint, with no swelling or marked tenderness. If you do attempt this exercise before you have sufficient strength in the joint, you will aggravate your symptoms.

Tip-Toe Through the Tulips

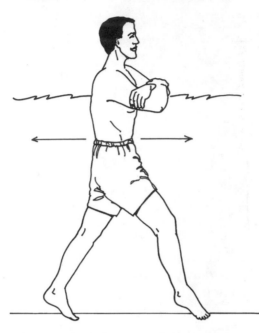

Position: Stand in chest-high water with your arms crossed over your chest.

Description: Walk on tip-toes only across the pool then walk backward to your starting position, just as in the warm-up laps. Repeat over and back across the pool several times on tip-toes.

Note: The arms have been taken out of this exercise to recruit the trunk for balancing and moving dynamically against resistance. By walking on tip-toes, you also make the base less stable, thus requiring more control and power from the legs and trunk. This exercise is excellent for dancers, or any athlete who plays a sport requiring exceptionally strong ankles—soccer, figure skating, hockey, and so on.

Precautions: None. Just make sure you have the arch and calf strength and endurance to do this exercise. Avoid it if you have any acute plantar fasciitis or Achilles tendinitis (refer to chapter 7).

Advanced Note: Remember to tighten your abdominals, low back, and buttocks to help stabilize the trunk and provide a solid base from which to move.

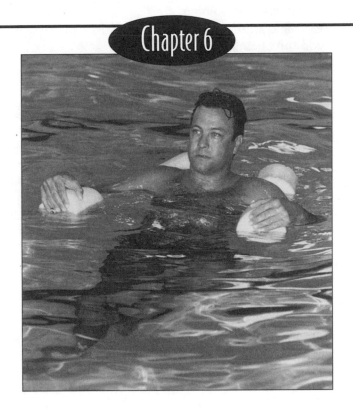

Deep Water Exercises

Endurance is vitally important to any fitness or rehabilitative program. You cannot safely progress to a more demanding and challenging workout level if you do not have a good foundation of endurance. You need stamina to stick with your exercise program and keep from tiring or sustaining injuries. Endurance is also crucial to building strength. One of the best ways to build endurance is through aerobic conditioning. Aerobic fitness and conditioning, which increase the efficiency of your heart, lungs, and blood, boost tissue healing as well.

Deep water exercises involve water running and jogging and are designed to build endurance. This occurs when you can do a demanding, sustained activity with little or no rest during the exercise. By using deep water in your exercise or therapeutic program, you get:

- increased cardiovascular training,
- increased overall endurance,
- full body workout against resistance,
- elimination of up to 90% or more of body weight,
- approximately 4 times more resistance working in a vertical position versus a horizontal position, and
- decreased compressive forces on the joints and discs of the spine.

Deep water exercise is important to the overall water therapy program. In the other portions of this program, you learned how to address flexibility, strength, and some coordination. Deep water exercise focuses on endurance and coordination. While water jogging or running, you are coordinating upper extremity and lower extremity movement patterns. You may also be incorporating diagonal patterns that allow you to move through several planes of motion.

Performing the deep water jogging at the end of the workout enables the muscles, joints, and tendons to open up joint spaces and enjoy a sustained, lengthening stretch overall. In working against the resistance of the water with the equipment planned as part of this program, the muscles and tendons go through repeated muscle shortening or contractions. Now that you have effectively worked the muscles, tendons, and ligaments, you can let them enjoy a subtle, sustained traction or elongating force in the deep water. In the deeper water, you also eliminate the compressive forces on the joints and spinal discs that result from the weight of the body. If you are experiencing pain prior to exercising, you can take advantage of the properties of the deep water to decrease the pain and enable you to exercise more comfortably.

Because you will be in deep water, you'll need to use some sort of flotation device. The Aquajogger belt is ideal, but a wide ski belt will work too. The beauty of the belt, and its main purpose, is to foster and maintain a neutral spinal alignment. You will be leaning slightly forward in your deep water work. Look at the illustrations on the following pages and notice the entire body is inclined slightly forward. There is no bending at the waist—you must maintain an erect posture. Also, big arm swings or pumping motions with the elbows result in trunk rotation and stabilization with the abdominal muscles. You can't miss with the deep water—everything is working hard, with no jarring or weightbearing.

It is in your best interest to include deep water jogging in your water therapy program. The benefits are undeniable, and it's fun! Invest in some deep water gear today!

The exercises and the pages on which they appear follow.

Deep Water Jogging

Position: Aquajogger (or ski belt) is secured tightly around the waist. Get in a depth of water where you are unable to touch the floor. If you don't want to get completely in the deep end, get where you can just touch bottom with your toes.

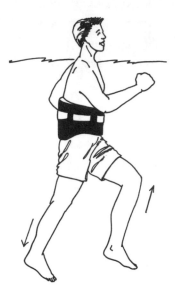

Description: Lean slightly forward while maintaining an erect posture just like the illustration. Bicycle with the legs while swinging the elbows in a pumping motion. Elbows are bent at a 90-degree angle. Start with forearms at waist level and push up toward the water's surface while bicycling with legs. Head and eyes are looking straight ahead. Jog nonstop, to your tolerance. Start with about 7 minutes and add a little more each time.

Note: Be sure the whole body is on a slightly forward lean, and that you are not bending forward from the hips. Remember to straighten your leg out completely as you go across the pool.

Precautions: None, really. If this exercise bothers your neck, relax your arm swing to a slower, longer, and more fluid motion instead of a pumping action.

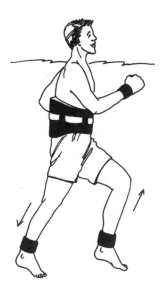

Variation: Advanced levels can use aqua shoes for additional resistance to the legs. Also, ankle weights can be used, with 1-5 lbs. (maximum) sufficient. For upper extremity resistance, use webbed gloves or wrist weights 1-1.5 lbs. (maximum). Do not add heavy weights because that will stress the shoulder or hip joints.

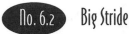 **Big Stride**

Position: Aquajogger (or ski belt) is secured tightly around the waist. Get in a depth of water where you are unable to touch the floor, or just touch with your tip-toes.

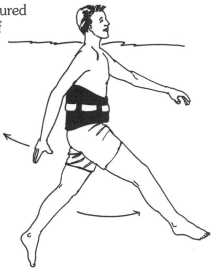

Description: Lean slightly forward while maintaining an erect position. The elbows and knees are locked—no bending of the limbs in this exercise. Swing the opposite arm and leg forward in an exaggerated stride and repeat with other side. Pull the foot up tight (instead of pointing it) to tighten the thigh muscles—the quadriceps. The motion resembles a stiff-legged march. Repeat 20-30 times, or do big strides 1-2 minutes without stopping.

Note: As you gain endurance, and you find you like this particular move, do it for a longer period of time, or alternate it with Aquajogging as a resting move. Of course, the faster your stride, the greater the resistance.

Precautions: None. If this makes your low back uncomfortable, shorten your stride and arm swings.

Variation: Advanced levels can add aqua shoes or light weights for additional resistance. Add light ankle weights (1-3 lbs. maximum) or even aqua shoes for lower extremity resistance. Add light wrist weights (1-1.5 lbs.) or use the hand barbells for added upper extremity resistance. Do the exaggerated striding of the soldier. Repeat 30 or more times, or do 1-3 minutes without stopping. This is a good warm-up or cool-down exercise.

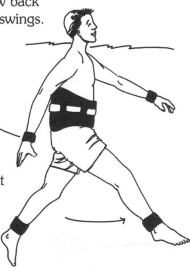

Note: If you speed up your moves, shorten the stride because of the added resistance.

No. 6.3 Jumping Jacks

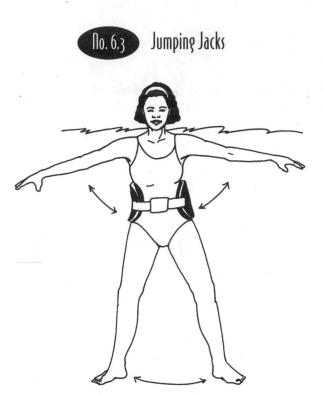

Position: An Aquajogger (or ski belt) is secured tightly around the waist. Get in a depth of water where you are unable to touch the floor.

Description: Start with your legs together and your arms against the trunk. Now, just like in physical education classes, press arms up to surface of water, and push legs open. You are not doing anything special with the hands here—just do those underwater jumping jacks without breaking the surface of the water. Repeat 20-30 times, or do for 1-2 minutes without stopping.

Note: If you start bobbing too much, shorten the arm movements. Do this before or after your water jogging; do it as an exercise. The water jogging should be done for an extended period of time without stopping to build endurance. Do this exercise to work different muscles, but do it for 1-3 minutes without stopping. This is a good exercise to do while you talk to your workout partner.

Precautions: None. If you have had a total hip replacement, do not cross the mid-line of the body (as in a scissoring motion).

Deep Water Abs

Equipment: Use your hand barbells or large floating barbells to help maintain balance and control in this exercise.

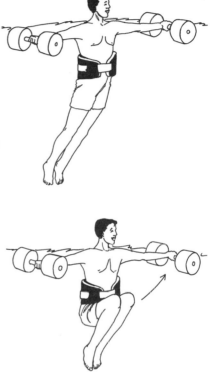

Position: An Aquajogger (or ski belt) is secured tightly around the waist. Get in a depth of water where you are unable to touch the floor. You may hold on to the side of the pool, or use barbell floats or kickboards to hold on to while exercising.

Description: Pull the knees up toward the chest and relax down. Now, pull the knees to the right of the chest and relax down. Pull knees up to the chest at midline and relax down. Repeat the movement to the left side of the chest and relax down. It will be a 1-2-3-4 motion. 1) Pull knees up to chest at midline and relax; 2) pull knees up to the right of the chest and relax down; 3) pull knees up and relax; 4) pull knees to the left and relax.

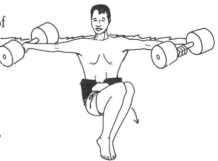

Note: By pulling up to the midline, then to both the right and left sides of the chest, you work the entire abdominal musculature. Repeat 30 times, or do this for 1-2 minutes without stopping.

Precautions: None. Keep your knees together and twist at the waist, not at the hip joint.

Part III

Programs for Common Injuries

The third part of *Water Exercise* is devoted entirely to common injuries or surgeries to specific joints or areas and their rehabilitation through water exercise. A therapeutic exercise program was designed for each specific injury or surgery starting with the beginner level, progressing to the intermediate level, and concluding with the advanced water exercises. The water exercise program incorporates necessary precautions and therapeutic goals for specific injuries or surgeries that are standard protocol in the clinical setting.

The difference between land-based and water-based exercises is the enhanced overall movement and reduction of pain in water. This is discussed in chapter 1 of this book. Pain management can be a major obstacle in the recovery process. The properties of water allow for better pain control. It is an appropriate alternative to the clinical setting when the individual simply is sidelined by pain and cannot participate effectively in his or her rehabilitation.

Each chapter in Part III covers a specific joint or body area and the most common injuries or surgeries to that area. Chapter 7 covers the lower leg, ankle, and foot; chapter 8 covers the knee; chapter 9 details the thigh, pelvis, and hip; chapter 10 details the trunk and spine and their common injuries; chapter 11 covers the shoulder; and chapter 12 details injuries common to the lower arm and wrist.

In each chapter, a specific water exercise program is detailed in the beginner, intermediate, and advanced levels and references the exercises presented in Part II of the book. For example, the knee has High Kicks in the beginner level listed as #3.3. That means it is the third exercise listed in the third chapter. The advanced program for the knee lists Hip In and Outs as an exercise, and is denoted as #5.5. That means this particular advanced exercise is the fifth exercise listed in chapter 5. Chapter 3 has the beginner level, chapter 4 the intermediate level, and chapter 5 the advanced level of exercises. We refer to the different levels of exercise programs in the injury-specific chapters for ease in locating the exercise in Part II of the book if necessary.

There is information on each injury or surgery in the respective chapters in Part III to provide you with a better understanding of the mechanisms of injury and the goals of rehabilitation.

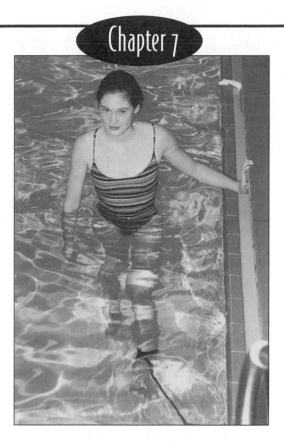

Lower Leg, Ankle, and Foot

Chapter 7 specifically outlines the causes and effects of plantar fascitis, Achilles tendinitis, ankle sprains, and lower leg and foot stress fractures.

Most of these injuries result from chronic overuse during specific sports activities. Some of the overuse injuries come from muscle imbalances. One muscle is consistently used more than another, resulting in respective overdevelopment and underdevelopment between the two muscle groups. This imbalance sets up the individual for a potential injury. Through the use of water exercise, muscle imbalances can be addressed and weaker areas developed to lend a broader base of support to the joint.

The lower leg takes a lot of abuse due to the highly repetitive nature of many sports. Muscle imbalances can also develop because of flattened or unusually high arches. Cross-training or rehabilitation creates a more proportionate base of strength between all the involved muscles.

Each injury is discussed, followed by an appropriate water therapy exercise program from the beginner, intermediate, and advanced levels of difficulty. This progression through the stages of recovery allows for comprehensive healing and protection of the weakened area from the possibility of reinjury.

PLANTAR FASCITIS

The muscle that flexes the toes of the foot, the plantaris, originates on the underside of the heel. Acute strain of this muscle and surrounding tissue is known as plantar fascitis. It is a condition aggravated by weightbearing and relieved by non-weightbearing. Full weightbearing means there is no use of assistive walking devices such as a cane, crutches, or walker. Non-weightbearing means the doctor has given specific instructions to place no weight at all on the involved leg or foot. Acute strain to the plantar fascia can result from muscle imbalance, a flattened arch, a high arch, and repetitive weightbearing with extension of the toes, as in running. Many people experience acute plantar fascitis when they start a new exercise program or suddenly increase their running distance. Strain can also occur when moving from a rigid shoe to a soft flexible shoe or, with women, when going from high heels to flat shoes. This causes the plantaris to suddenly lengthen. Strengthening of the foot, arch, and ankle musculature corrects plantar fascitis. In addition, the use of a small heel lift is helpful during the early acute phase when the area is tender and inflamed.

ACHILLES TENDINITIS

Achilles tendinitis is the inflammation of the Achilles tendon, the strong band that runs behind the ankle and attaches into the heel. Achilles tendinitis is not unlike plantar fascitis and is caused by similar conditions. Muscle imbalances and inflexibility of the gastrocnemius (calf muscle) quickly result in strain to the Achilles tendon. This injury may occur in running sports as well as jumping sports, including basketball, track, volleyball, and dance. Initially, rest and ice applied to the area are necessary. Once inflammation is down, strengthening of ankle musculature to correct the imbalance can begin. Stretching is essential in resolving Achilles tendinitis. Water is an excellent medium for rehabilitation because one is partially to completely non-weightbearing.

ANKLE SPRAINS

Ankle sprains are a common occurrence in sports. This injury usually results when one lands on the outside (lateral) portion of the foot and the angle and weight of the body force the foot sharply inward. There is diffuse tearing of tissue and, sometimes, ligaments. For this reason, ankle sprains should always be examined by a doctor, athletic trainer, or physical therapist to determine the extent of the injury. Rest off the foot, along with round-the-clock icing, is necessary during the first 2-3 days after injury. When cleared by your health care professional for rehabilitation, strengthening in all planes of movement is necessary to correct muscle imbalances and prevent recurrent sprains. Water is a perfect place to begin bearing weight again, which can be graduated from slight weightbearing to full weightbearing by moving from deep to shallow water. The ankle must be strengthened in both forward and backward motions, as well as side-to-side movements to *fully* rehabilitate it and guard against further injury. Switching to a high-top tennis shoe adds additional stability to the ankle for those individuals who are prone to recurrent sprains.

TIBIAL AND FIBULAR FRACTURES

Tibial fractures are less common than fibular fractures and usually result from trauma or vehicular accidents. The fibula, the smaller long bone of the lower extremity, is frequently fractured in skiing accidents, falls, or highly demanding sports such as long distance running or ballet. In most cases, casting and non-weightbearing are necessary for anywhere from 3 to 6 weeks. After clearance by a doctor, the initiation of gradual weightbearing begins, and the pool is the perfect place to start. One will begin in deeper water (chest high) and start with forward and backward movement patterns. As the healing continues, side-to-side movements are introduced. Next, one moves to shallower water to increase weightbearing on the lower extremity. By using the water, one encounters less pain and stiffness and can progress faster through the therapeutic program. In the initial phase of rehabilitation of a tibial or fibular fracture, water is ideal.

STRESS FRACTURES

Stress fractures occur in highly demanding, repetitive activities such as dance, running, basketball, and gymnastics. They occur when there is a biomechanical compromise, such as a flattened or extremely high arch, recurrent tendinitis, or muscle imbalance. Stress fractures can be hard to detect and may require more than one series of x-rays before a diagnosis can be made.

As mentioned in other conditions of the lower leg, rest and reintroduction of weightbearing to the area are necessary for complete healing. Flexibility must be reestablished before strengthening and endurance can occur. Always strengthen the area about the fracture site in all directions—forward, backward, and side-to-side. Weightbearing can be varied and increased in water by changing the depth in which one performs the therapeutic exercises.

EXERCISE PROGRAMS

The following exercise programs are designed to aid in the rehabilitation of the lower leg, ankle, and foot. Determine your exercise level based on the criteria presented in chapter 1. Then perform each listed exercise as instructed. Exercise numbers are included for quick reference.

Beginner Level

Perform one set of 15 repetitions in chest-high water for 2-3 weeks.

No. 3.1 Warm-Up Laps   26
No. 3.3 High Kicks   28

No. 3.4 Hip In and Outs   29
No. 3.26 Heel Rock and Rolls   51
No. 3.16 Squats—Double   41
No. 3.18 Ankle Inversion (isometric)   43
No. 3.19 Ankle Eversion (isometric)   44
No. 3.20 Hip Abduction Facing Wall   45
No. 3.10 Trunk Twists   35
No. 3.22 Scooter   47
No. 6.1 Deep Water Jogging (10-15 min.)   108
Sidestroke (both sides of the body) up to 10 min.

Intermediate Level

Do two sets of 15 repetitions in above-waist-high water for 3 to 6 weeks.

No. 3.1 Warm-Up Laps (Beginning)   26
No. 3.2 Sideways Walk   27
No. 3.3 High Kicks (Beginning)   28
No. 3.4 Hip In and Outs (Beginning)   29
No. 3.26 Heel Rock and Rolls   51
No. 3.16 Squats—Double   41
No. 3.18 Ankle Inversion (isometric)   43
No. 3.19 Ankle Eversion (isometric)   44
No. 4.25 Lateral Step-Ups   80
No. 5.18 Tip-Toe Through the Tulips
              (alternate with Heel Walks)   104
No. 4.19 Heel Walks   74
No. 3.11 Marching in Place   36
No. 4.23 Hop Scotch (chest-high water)   78
No. 6.1 Deep Water Jogging (15-20 min.)   108
No. 4.26 One-Legged Stork   81
No. 4.27 Lunges (Intermediate)   82
Sidestroke 10-15 min. (both sides of the body)

Advanced Level

Perform two sets of 20 repetitions in waist-high water for 6 to 12 weeks.

No. 5.1 Warm-Up Laps (Advanced)   87

No. 5.2 Carioca (Advanced)   88

No. 5.4 High Kicks (Advanced)   90

No. 5.5 Hip In and Outs (Advanced)   91

No. 5.18 Tip-Toe Through the Tulips
          (alternate with Heel Walks)   104

No. 4.19 Heel Walks   74

No. 4.25 Lateral Step-Ups   80

No. 4.24 Bunny Hop   79

No. 3.18 Ankle Inversion   43

No. 3.19 Ankle Eversion   44

No. 5.3 Lunges (Advanced)   89

No. 5.17 Lower Extremity Squares   103

No. 5.9 Squats With Ball   95

No. 6.1 Deep Water Jogging (20 min.)   108

Kicking with Fin (flexible versus stiff, rigid, or oversized fins)

Swimming (any combination of strokes)

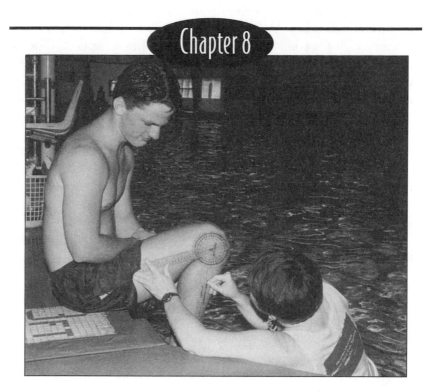

Chapter 8

Knee

The knee is one of the most complicated and vulnerable joints of the body. It is the connecting link and weightbearing joint between the hip and the foot. Many factors unrelated to the knee joint itself contribute to its potential for injury.

Angles play a major role in stress on the knee joint and can lead to degenerative changes over the years. For example, people who have knock-knees or bowed legs often develop knee problems later in life. Participation in sports further increases the chance for knee problems. Flattened or high arches, if they are extreme, are conditions that can place stress and strain on the joint surface of the knee. Someone who is bowlegged will experience more wear and tear on the inside of the joint surface, while someone who is knock-kneed will experience more degenerative changes on the outside surface of the knee joint over the years.

The knee is vulnerable to injury due to the demands of sports such as skiing, basketball, running, and soccer, to name a few. The nature of these sports calls for sudden stops and starts at higher speeds. They also require the individual to be able to move forward, backward, side-to-side, or any combination of these directions with split-second timing. Cross-training or rehabilitation to equally develop all the muscle groups surrounding the knee joint is key to recovery and injury prevention.

In this chapter, we discuss the mechanism of injury followed by a specific water exercise program covering beginner, intermediate, and advanced levels. Progressing through these stages of rehabilitation allows for proper healing and prevention of reinjury of the weakened area. Water is an excellent avenue of rehabilitation for knee injuries or following knee surgery because of the decreased compressive forces to the joint. Also, any injury to the knee is extremely painful and potentially disabling, so effective pain management is important to the recovery process.

The injuries and surgeries covered in chapter 8 include medial collateral sprains, chondromalacia (patellar problems), patellar (kneecap) dislocation, osteoarthritis, and anterior cruciate ligament reconstruction. Following the discussion of each injury is a water exercise program from beginner, intermediate, and advanced levels. A number denotes where the exercise is located in the book so you can refer to it. For example, No. 4.7 means the exercise is the seventh illustration in chapter 4. No. 3.15 means the exercise is in the third chapter and is the fifteenth illustration. Chapter 3 covers beginner, chapter 4 intermediate, and chapter 5 advanced exercises.

Please follow the program closely through the three stages of progression. Ideally, you should be consulting with your doctor or therapist when dealing with the knee joint. It is very vulnerable to both injury and reinjury, even through the rehabilitative process. Go slowly, according to the pace set by your doctor or therapist. You do not want to complicate and prolong your recovery from a knee injury or surgery by overdoing it. Comply with the specifics of the recovery program and its progression through the beginner, intermediate, and advanced exercises.

MEDIAL COLLATERAL LIGAMENTOUS SPRAIN

Medial collateral ligamentous sprain is one of the most common knee injuries and happens in all ages and classifications of athletes. The injury usually results from a direct blow to the outside of the knee that occurs in such sports as football or rugby. In other instances, the sprain happens when a sharp turn to the inside is made, as in a cutting move in the sports of skiing and soccer. Usually the athlete is trying to decelerate (slow down) when making the inside "cut." In all scenarios, the foot is planted and stable.

The sprain is classified as a first, second, or third degree sprain. In all instances, **R**est, **I**ce, **C**ompression, and **E**levation (R-I-C-E) are warranted for the first 48-72 hours. In second and third degree sprains, one is unable to completely straighten the leg and crutches are necessary to unload the joint and ligament from normal stresses and loads in order for healing to occur. The more severe the sprain, the more disabling the symptoms, with a third degree sprain being the most involved. There is a complete loss of joint stability and possible accompanying injury to the anterior cruciate ligament in third degree sprains. Water therapy is an excellent mode of rehabilitation for medial collateral sprains due to the gravity-free environment. There is little compressive joint force from weightbearing and the weight of the leg is buttressed through the buoyancy of the water. Initially, flexion of the knee (bending with weightbearing) is avoided. The focus of the rehabilitation is the strengthening and flexibility of all the muscle groups that stabilize the knee, and those involved with the ankle and hip joints.

CHONDROMALACIA

Chondromalacia of the knee is common among teenagers, young adults, and runners. It manifests as a grinding sensation under the kneecap and is aggravated with activities requiring repetitive flexion and extension (bending and straightening) of the knee. Walking, ballet, running, squatting, or frequently going up and down stairs may lead to chondromalacia. This syndrome is painful due to the gradual erosion of the articulating surface on the underside of the patella. In athletes, chondromalacia consistently appears after running a set distance, usually about 2 miles, before the pain becomes unbearable and they must stop.

Specific causes of chondromalacia are unknown. However, it is felt that a number of things contribute, including some structural or biomechanical dysfunction that interrupts the normal rhythm of the patellar tracking. Dysfunctional biomechanical factors could include flat arches, unusually high arches, bowlegged or knock-kneed posture, weak quadriceps (anterior thigh) or tight hamstrings (posterior thigh).

Rehabilitation should focus on strengthening all the stabilizing muscles of the knee—inner and outer thigh, and the anterior and posterior thigh (quadriceps and hamstrings). Somewhere there is a muscle or structural imbalance that has contributed to the chondromalacia.

Water exercise can easily accommodate lower extremity strengthening in an unloaded environment to lessen the knee joint compressive forces.

PATELLAR SUBLUXATION OR DISLOCATION

Patellar subluxation or dislocation may be a one-time incident or recurrent in nature. The instability may be related to a number of conditions that include knock-kneed posture, weak quadriceps, ligament laxity, flattened arches, or patellar misalignment, where the patella is located outward of the midline of the knee.

Patellar subluxation related to sports usually occurs when the foot is planted and a sharp inside move is made. The weak inner quadriceps muscle is unable to stabilize the patella and it subluxes or dislocates laterally (outside) of its bony groove. If the patella completely dislocates out of its tracking groove, it must be mobilized back in place by the physician or athletic trainer as soon as possible. R-I-C-E: **R**est, **I**ce, **C**ompression, and **E**levation follow, with further diagnostic evaluation recommended.

As in other conditions of the injured knee, all muscle groups involved in knee stabilization must be strengthened so muscle imbalances are corrected. A knee support with a horseshoe-shaped pad is helpful for recurrent patellar subluxation. Ask your doctor, physical therapist, or athletic trainer if this would be helpful in your particular case. Water exercise is an excellent medium to facilitate the return to sports through a safe, controlled environment.

OSTEOARTHRITIS OF THE KNEE

Osteoarthritis of the knee is not uncommon and results from cumulative major and microtraumas over the years. Degenerative changes result from uneven weightbearing from meniscal tears, leg-length disparity, and knock-kneed or bowlegged knees. Carrying additional weight over the years also contributes to degenerative changes. Conservative treatment through physical therapy includes heat, ultrasound, and strengthening exercises. Anti-inflammatory medications and weight loss help ease the pain, but ultimately joint replacement surgery is the most effective means of managing degenerative arthritis of the knee.

Water exercise is a very effective and comfortable way to manage degenerative arthritis of the knee, whether one has had surgery or is trying to prevent it. The gravity-free environment of the water reduces compressive joint forces while one works on strength and endurance. Water is helpful in the management of arthritic pain but it cannot reverse degenerative processes.

ANTERIOR CRUCIATE LIGAMENT RECONSTRUCTION

Anterior cruciate ligament reconstruction is a memorable process—akin to childbirth according to many women patients! This is the most commonly disrupted ligament of the knee, and also the most disabling. The knee is most vulnerable when the foot is planted and the lower leg is rotated. This injury commonly occurs in sports in which stop-start motions with cutting movements are involved, such as soccer or football. Skiing is another sport where injuries to the anterior cruciate ligament are common.

When this injury occurs, there is usually an audible pop followed by immediate disabling pain and an inability to walk unassisted or to fully extend the leg. Medically, it is felt this injury is best treated through surgery, unless the patient is not very active or plans to modify his or her lifestyle. Sometimes a good strengthening program and lifestyle modification suffice. However, further injury or complete tearing of the ligament is not that uncommon down the road.

Water exercise is an excellent way to rehabilitate this injury owing to the ability to get started soon after surgery. Weightbearing can be graduated in the water as the individual progresses through the various stages of rehabilitation. The doctor, physical therapist, or athletic trainer can guide you through the appropriate levels. Please adhere to their parameters closely to ensure proper healing. Through water, rehabilitation from anterior cruciate ligament reconstruction is less painful, highly effective, and comprehensive.

EXERCISE PROGRAMS

The following exercise programs are designed to aid in the rehabilitation of the knee. Determine your exercise level based on the criteria presented in chapter 1. Perform each exercise listed as instructed. Exercise numbers are included for quick reference.

Beginner Level

Perform one set of 10-15 repetitions, and continue at this level for 3 to 4 weeks.

No. 3.1 Warm-Up Laps   26
No. 3.2 Sideways Walk   27
No. 3.26 Heel Rock and Rolls   51
No. 3.20 Hip Abduction Facing Wall   45
No. 3.3 High Kicks (*with bent leg)   28
No. 3.10 Trunk Twists   35
No. 3.15 Bird   40
No. 3.14 Gorilla Press-Downs   39
No. 3.7 Chest Flys   32
No. 3.11 Marching in Place   36
No. 4.26 One-Legged Stork   81
*With/without brace, according to your doctor or physical therapist.

Intermediate Level

Perform two sets of 15 repetitions, and continue at this level for 4 weeks, or according to your doctor's or physical therapist's guidelines.

No. 3.1 Warm-Up Laps (Beginning)   26
No. 3.2 Sideways Walk   27
Continue with Beginner Level exercises and increase repetitions.
No. 3.3 High Kicks (Beginning; with straight leg)   28
No. 3.4 Hip In and Outs (Beginning)   29
No. 3.24 Adductor Squeezes   49

No. 3.16 Squats—Double   41

No. 3.22 Scooter   47

No. 4.28 Sitting Abdominal and Hip Crunches   83

No. 6.1 Deep Water Jogging (8-15 min., to tolerance)   108

Advanced Level

Perform three sets of 15 repetitions, and continue at this level for 4-6 weeks, or according to your doctor's or physical therapist's guidelines.

No. 5.1 Warm-Up Laps (Advanced)   87

No. 5.2 Carioca (Advanced)   88

Continue with previous Beginner Level and Intermediate Level exercises as designated.

No. 4.14 Hip Extension With Cords (Pull-Backs)   69

No. 4.15 Hip Flexion With Cords (Pull-Forwards)   70

No. 4.16 Hip Abduction With Cords (Pull-Outs)   71

No. 4.17 Hip Adduction With Cords (Pull-Ins)   72

No. 3.21 Figure 8   46

No. 4.25 Lateral Step-Ups   80

No. 4.24 Bunny Hop   79

No. 6.1 Deep Water Jogging (15-20 min., or to tolerance)   108

No. 5.3 Lunges (Advanced)   89

No. 5.9 Squats With Ball   5

Flutter Kicking—as indicated by your doctor or physical therapist

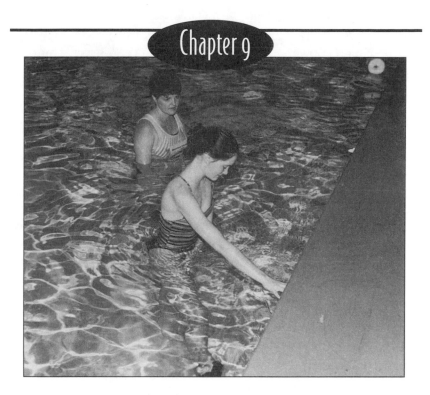

Chapter 9

Thigh, Pelvis, and Hip

In this chapter, we cover some common injuries to the thigh, pelvis, and hip areas. Many of these are muscular strain injuries that can occur from overuse or inflexibility.

All of the injuries covered in this chapter involve muscle groups with attachments to the pelvis. The hamstrings, quadriceps, and adductor muscle groups all work in relation to the hip and knee, and to the placement of the leg in space. Muscle strains of the thigh and hip are common in sports that involve jumping, running, side-to-side movements, and sudden stopping and starting. Such injuries are found primarily in basketball, volleyball, track, dance, tennis, and soccer. The muscles involved include the quadriceps (front thigh), hamstrings (posterior thigh), adductors (inner thigh), hip flexors (groin area), and hip extensors (gluteal or buttock muscles). Explosive movements from a stationary position or a sudden movement to change direction can strain any one or combination of the above muscles. Unfortunately, these injuries are not easily resolved and can be recurrent in nature if one returns to full activity before the area has had time to heal properly. The healing phase may take anywhere from 1 month to an entire sport's season.

Also discussed in this chapter is osteoarthritis of the hip. This is a condition that results from wear and tear on the joint over the years and may be related to a congenital condition, leg-length difference, or trauma. Degenerative changes result from unequal weightbearing on the hip joint surface.

Each condition or injury discussion is followed by a water exercise program covering the beginner, intermediate, and advanced levels of difficulty. For ease of reference, each exercise is preceded by a number, such as No. 3.7, which means this particular exercise is located in chapter 3 and is the seventh illustration. Chapter 3 covers the beginner level, chapter 4 covers the intermediate level, and chapter 5 covers the advanced level of exercises.

HAMSTRING STRAIN

Hamstring strain is an injury common to all sports. The strain may range in severity from minor soreness of the muscle belly in the posterior thigh to actual rupture of the muscle belly with hemorrhaging (deep bruising and bleeding). Hamstring strain is prevalent in track, football, and soccer due to the explosive demands of these sports.

QUADRICEPS STRAIN

Quadriceps strain is similar in characteristics to hamstring strain. It occurs more often in jumping sports or in soccer when a sudden, forceful contraction of the muscle is necessary to kick the ball. It ranges from minor strains that heal with 2-3 days of rest to the actual rupture of the quadriceps muscle. There may be little bruising of the frontal thigh, but marked tenderness and muscle spasm are common. The quadriceps are actually four different muscles that extend or straighten the lower leg. Marked quadriceps development occurs as a result of repetitive knee extension particularly among competitive athletes who participate in soccer, swimming, tennis, and running.

ADDUCTOR STRAIN

Adductor strain, an injury to the inner thigh muscles, occurs in those athletes whose sport requires repetitive side-to-side movement with sudden stops and starts. These would include soccer, tennis, basketball, football, and racquetball. Injury to this muscle group and/or the hip flexors is referred to as a groin injury. Groin strains can occur in hockey, gymnastics, and baseball as well. Groin strains do require rest and can be slow to heal in general.

HIP POINTER

Hip pointer injuries primarily occur in contact sports such as football or rugby and are quite painful initially. The injury occurs when a blow is taken on the front portion of the hip and slightly below the waist in the area know as the iliac crest. After a direct blow to this area, an athlete may experience immediate pain and spasm as well as an inability to rotate the trunk or flex the leg (*Modern Principles of Athletic Training*, D. Arnheim). An exam by a physician is mandatory to rule out fracture or structural damage to the iliac crest.

All strains require R-I-C-E initially: **R**est, **I**ce, **C**ompression, and **E**levation.

EXERCISE PROGRAMS

The following exercise programs are designed to aid in the rehabilitation of the thigh, pelvis, and hip. Determine your exercise level based on the criteria presented in chapter 1. Then perform each exercise listed as instructed. Exercise numbers are included for quick reference.

Beginner Level

During the first 72 hours after injury

Rest—from the sport or other activity;

Ice—to injured muscle group throughout the day;

Compression—by Ace bandage or elastic support to injured muscle group; and

Elevation—stay off the feet as much as possible.

After 72 hours and clearance by the doctor, physical therapist, or athletic trainer, start a gentle stretching and range-of-motion program and continue for the next 4-6 days.

No. 3.1 Warm-Up Laps (chest-high water)   26

No. 3.2 Sideways Walk (chest-high water)   27

No. 3.24 Adductor Squeezes —10 repetitions   49

No. 4.26 One-Legged Stork—10 repetitions, alternating legs   81

No. 6.1 Deep Water Jogging—10-15 min. maximum   108

Intermediate Level

After 10 days to 4 weeks following injury, perform two sets of 10-12 repetitions.

No. 3.1 Warm-Up Laps (Beginning)   26

No. 3.2 Sideways Walk (chest-high water)   27

No. 3.3 High Kicks (Beginning)   28

No. 3.20 Hip Abduction Facing Wall   45

No. 3.26 Heel Rock and Rolls   51

No. 3.16 Squats—Double (above-the-waist water)   41

No. 3.21 Figure 8   46

No. 4.21 Lateral Trunk Flexion (Hula Dancer)   76

No. 3.12 Knee to Chest (Hip Flexion)   37

No. 6.1 Deep Water Jogging (15-20 min.)   108

Flutter Kicking (5-10 min.)

Advanced Level

One month after injury or pain-free range of motion, perform two sets of 15 repetitions and continue for 4 to 8 weeks.

No. 5.1 Warm-Up Laps (Advanced)   87

No. 5.2 Carioca (Advanced)   88

No. 5.4 High Kicks (Advanced)   90

No. 5.5 Hip In and Outs (Advanced)   91

No. 5.9 Squats With Ball   95

No. 5.3 Lunges (Advanced)   89

No. 4.24 Bunny Hop (chest-high water)   79

No. 5.17 Lower Extremity Squares (chest-high water)   103

No. 4.25 Lateral Step-Ups   80

No. 4.28 Sitting Abdominal and Hip Crunches   83

No. 6.1 Deep Water Jogging (20 min.)   108

Sidestroke, freestyle, or backstroke with fins (10-15 min.)

Add gradual increments of activity starting with a walk/jog of 1-2 miles, then increasing to jogging only from 1-3 miles. When you can do this without pain or development of symptoms, gradually begin resumption of the sport. Work with an athletic trainer, physical therapist, or doctor in this phase if at all possible.

OSTEOARTHRITIS OF THE HIP

Osteoarthritis, degenerative changes of the hip, commonly appear in both sexes at around 50 years of age. Degenerative changes can occur in the hip joint in the articulating cartilage or as a result of congenital conditions. They may also occur from joint disease, trauma, repeated episodes of inflammatory arthritis (rheumatoid), or lifelong wear and tear as a result of a leg-length disparity.

The degenerative process is insidious and may appear as generalized hip pain or stiffness, especially in the morning. Pain is worse with weightbearing; the longer one is up the worse the pain gets as the day goes on. Rest brings relief. Daily activities such as putting on socks and shoes or pants become more difficult. Stiffness and gradual loss of range of motion result in shortened stride and difficulties in walking. Eventually, a cane may be needed to assist in walking. Getting up and down as well as climbing stairs becomes particularly painful and difficult. Ultimately, surgery in the form of a total hip replacement is the most effective management of osteoarthritis of the hip. With surgery, the individual can continue a productive lifestyle with no loss of functional ability to perform daily activities.

Water exercise is excellent for the surgically or non-surgically treated arthritic hip. Water offers a gravity-eliminated environment with reduced compressive forces on the joints, variable weightbearing according to the depth of the water, and additional support through buoyancy. The following program is appropriate for both the non-operated-on hip and total replacement hip. All total hip replacement patients must have clearance by their physicians before starting any exercise program.

Beginner Level

Wait 8-12 weeks after surgery as indicated by your physician or physical therapist. Follow the program for 3-4 weeks, performing 3-4 times a week only. Do one set of 15 repetitions.

No. 3.1 Warm-Up Laps (chest-high water)   26

No. 3.2 Sideways Walk (chest-high water)   27

No. 3.26 Heel Rock and Rolls   51

No. 3.3 High Kicks (no backward motion)   28
Remember these precautions: Do not kick higher than a 90-degree angle and do not cross the midline (middle) of the body. Talk to your doctor or physical therapist if you have any questions.

No. 3.16 Squats—Double (chest-high water; half knee bends only!)   41

No. 3.5 Abdominal Press-Downs   30

No. 3.14 Gorilla Press-Downs   39

No. 3.15 Bird   40

No. 3.20 Hip Abduction Facing Wall   45

No. 4.26 One-Legged Stork (alternate legs)   81

No. 6.1 Deep Water Jogging (8-12 min.)   108

Intermediate Level

After 3-4 weeks at the Beginner Level, move to the Intermediate Level. Perform two sets of 10-12 repetitions, and stay at this level for 2-3 weeks.

No. 3.1 Warm-Up Laps (Beginning)   26
No. 3.2 Sideways Walk   27

Continue with Beginner Level exercises and increase repetitions. Add the following to the program:

No. 3.22 Scooter   47
No. 6.1 Deep Water Jogging (20 min.)   108
No. 3.7 Chest Flys   32
No. 3.8 Shoulder Press-Downs   33
No. 3.24 Adductor Squeezes   49

Advanced Level

Perform two sets of 15 repetitions, then progress to Advanced Level after 2-3 weeks in the Intermediate phase.

No. 5.1 Warm-Up Laps (Advanced)   87
No. 3.2 Sideways Walk   27

Continue with previous exercises from the Beginner and Intermediate Levels. Add the following to the program:

No. 4.27 Lunges (Intermediate)   82
No. 5.9 Squats   95
No. 6.1 Deep Water Jogging (20 min.)   108
Flutter Kicking
Freestyle, Backstroke, or Sidestroke only

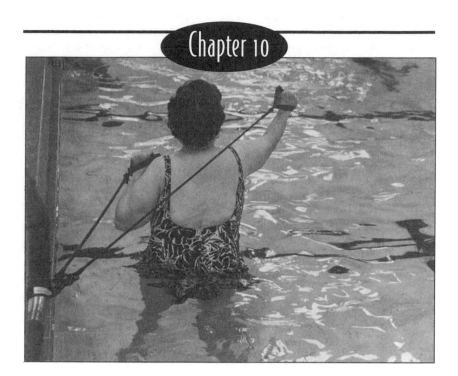

Chapter 10

Trunk and Spine

Statistics show that about 8 out of 10 individuals will suffer some type of low back pain or dysfunction in their lifetimes. Back pain can be as varied as those individuals suffering from it. The treatment of back pain remains ever-challenging for the medical profession because it must be considered on an individual basis. If someone has a broken arm or an ankle sprain, there are standard treatment protocols. However, when someone comes in with complaints of back pain, the doctor or therapist must rule out several possible causes of the pain to arrive at its origin. This process may involve more diagnostic measures, including x-rays, CT scans, or an MRI to arrive at a probable cause of pain.

The rehabilitation of the back is as varied as the many types of back pain. Because of this, chapter 10 on the trunk and spine is a bit different from the previous chapters. One exercise may be indicated for one type of back pain, yet should be avoided with another type of back pain. This chapter will address the following: chronic low back pain, spondylolysis, spondylolisthesis, and scoliosis. These conditions affect the skeletal system or the spine. Herniated and bulging discs, sometimes referred to as slipped discs, are addressed generally in the chronic back pain segment. However, due to the complexity and scope of this condition, it cannot be addressed adequately in one chapter.

A global program is presented in the beginner, intermediate, and advanced levels. The exercises included in the global section are appropriate and safe for *all* the back conditions covered in this chapter. Then, specific exercises that are appropriate and safe for each specific type of back condition are covered.

For example, if you have scoliosis that doesn't require surgery, you would follow the global program in the beginner, intermediate, and advanced levels and any exercises indicated under scoliosis. Again, it is important to follow the program *specific* to your back problem to effectively and safely rehabilitate your condition.

CHRONIC LOW BACK PAIN

Chronic low back pain is familiar to all of us, either on a firsthand basis or through a family member or co-worker. Most individuals with chronic back pain have run the medical gamut in the form of physical therapy, chiropractic, massage therapy, acupuncture, or management by pain medications. Most of these resulted in temporary relief at best because they are passive in nature. In other words, nothing is required on the part of the individual; he or she is totally dependent on the health care practitioner for the management or "cure" of the pain. Whether the chronicity of the back pain is from an unsuccessful surgery, faulty posture, or an untreated condition or accident, the individual must return to a consistent level of activity to combat the pain. The water is highly effective for back pain because of the unloading of the joints and discs inherent in a gravity-eliminated environment. The key to managing chronic back pain is the restoration of functional activity and motion.

SPONDYLOLYSIS

Spondylolysis is the degeneration and accompanying stress fracture or defect in the articulating processes of the vertebrae. It occurs in the lower lumbar spine, usually at the L4-L5 level. This condition, more common in males, may be congenital in nature or may occur in athletes of certain sports in which there is a high volume of certain movements, including hyperextension of the lumbar spine with excessive rotation. Such sports include gymnastics, ballet, butterfly stroke in swimming, spiking the volleyball, serving in tennis, or interior line blocking in football. Disc bulge or herniation may accompany this condition. Water therapy and fitness are conducive to rehabilitating spondylolysis because of the gravity-eliminated, little-to-no-weightbearing environment. All activities that increase weightbearing through the spine should be avoided, such as squats and lunges in weightlifting. Climbing stairs also increases the load on the spine. Avoid all hyperextension of the spine. In swimming, the backstroke, butterfly, and breaststroke hyperextend the spine— avoid them. The sidestroke is a safe and appropriate stroke for spondylolysis because it keeps the back in a neutral or protected position. Abdominal strengthening exercises are also excellent for spondylolysis. Avoid hyperextension of the back and activities that increase weightbearing through the spine with this particular back condition.

SPONDYLOLISTHESIS

Spondylolisthesis is the forward slippage of one vertebra onto the vertebra below it, most commonly at L4-L5. The condition may have evolved from unmanaged spondylolysis. Radiating pain into the buttocks or legs may occur from pressure on the nerve roots from the forward displacement of the vertebra onto the other. There are different stages of slippage and all are manageable; surgery is rarely necessary. Spondylolisthesis and spondylolysis are both detectable by x-ray. As with spondylolysis, hyperextension and loading of the spine should be avoided. Work from a neutral, protected position to strengthen the trunk. Abdominal strengthening exercises are indicated, as are any upright, sustained activities, such as water jogging.

SCOLIOSIS

Scoliosis is also known as curvature of the spine. In scoliosis, there is a lateral deviation from the midline of the back with a rotary component. Scoliosis is very manageable and primarily occurs in the thoracic and lumbar spine. The greater the lateral deviation, the greater rotation of the spine overall. Scoliosis may result in back spasms and sometimes disc compromise; surgery is required in cases of extreme curvature and rotation.

In unoperated scoliosis, we focus on strengthening the trunk as a whole, including back extensors and abdominals. Unilateral (one-sided) exercises are also included to strengthen the convex side (where the large curvature is located) and stretch the tightness of the concave side. In cases of scoliosis where surgery was necessary, the focus of the exercises is to strengthen and stabilize the trunk as a whole. Flexibility is easier to work on in water because of the non-weightbearing, buoyant environment.

EXERCISE PROGRAMS

The following exercises make up a global program with a focus on trunk strengthening and stabilization. They are safe and appropriate for all of the back conditions in this chapter. Determine your exercise level based on the criteria presented in chapter 1. Then perform the specific exercise as it is presented. Exercise numbers are included for quick reference.

If you have herniated disc(s), follow the beginner level program as presented. Do not add the additional exercises that are presented for the other back conditions. They are not appropriate for herniated disc conditions and they have the potential to aggravate symptoms.

Beginner Level

Perform one set of 15 to 20 repetitions.

No. 3.1 Warm-Up Laps   26
No. 3.2 Sideways Walk   27
No. 3.3 High Kicks   28

No. 3.20 Hip Abduction Facing Wall   45

No. 3.26 Heel Rock and Rolls   51

No. 3.24 Adductor Squeezes   49

No. 3.7 Chest Flys   32

No. 3.8 Shoulder Press-Downs   33

No. 3.14 Gorilla Press-Downs   39

No. 3.15 Bird   40

No. 3.25 Unloading the Spine (5-10 min.)   50

No. 6.1 Deep Water Jogging (deep end or chest-high water)   108

If you have chronic back pain, you may add the following exercises to your program.

No. 3.10 Trunk Twists   35

No. 3.4 Hip In and Outs   29

No. 3.16 Squats—Double   41

If you have spondylolysis or spondylolisthesis, add the following exercises to your program.

No. 3.13 Barbell Push-Pulls   38

No. 4.7 Side-Swipes With Paddle   62

Sidestroke only if swimming; avoid other strokes because they place the back in hyperextension.

If you have unoperated scoliosis, add the following exercises in addition to the beginner program.

No. 4.1 Alternate Press-Downs (with paddles)   56

No. 4.21 Lateral Trunk Flexion (Hula Dancer; both sides)   76

No. 4.7 Side-Swipes With Paddle (both sides)   62

Intermediate Exercises

Perform two sets of 15 repetitions. Continue the beginner level exercises as presented and increase the repetitions and sets as previously noted. Add these exercises as indicated.

No. 4.5 Upright Rows With Cords   60

No. 4.6 Punches With Cords   61

No. 3.5 Abdominal Press-Downs (Beginning)   30

No. 6.1 Deep Water Jogging (increase to 15-20 min.)   108

No. 4.7 Side-Swipes With Paddle   62

Sidestroke on both sides of the body to tolerance. Avoid other strokes at this point.

If you have chronic back pain, add these additional exercises to your intermediate program.

No. 4.20 Carioca (Intermediate)   75

No. 4.27 Lunges (Intermediate)   82

No. 4.28 Sitting Abdominal and Hip Crunches   83

No. 4.1 Alternate Press-Downs (with paddles)   56

If you have spondylolysis or spondylolisthesis, add these exercises to the global intermediate program.

No. 4.28 Sitting Abdominal and Hip Crunches   83

No. 4.1 Alternate Press-Downs (with paddles)   56

No. 3.16 Squats—Double (waist-high water)   41

If you have herniated discs, add the following exercises to the global intermediate program.

No. 4.1 Alternate Press-Downs (with paddles)   56

No. 4.27 Lunges (Intermediate; if there is no leg pain, i.e., radiating, sharp leg pain as opposed to muscle soreness)   82

If you have unoperated scoliosis, add the following exercises in addition to the intermediate global program.

No. 4.29 Windmills   84

No. 5.9 Squats With Ball   95

Advanced Level

Perform two sets of 20 repetitions.

No. 5.1 Warm-Up Laps (Advanced)   87

No. 5.2 Carioca (Advanced)   88

No. 5.9 Squats With Ball   95

No. 5.16 Seated Surfer 102

No. 5.11 Upper Extremity PNF Diagonal 97

No. 3.7 Chest Flys 32

No. 3.8 Shoulder Press-Downs 33

No. 4.1 Alternate Press-Downs 56

No. 4.7 Side-Swipes With Paddle 62

No. 3.15 Bird 40

No. 3.14 Gorilla Press-Downs 39

No. 3.13 Barbell Push-Pulls 38

No. 6.1 Deep Water Jogging (increase to 20-30 min.) 108

No. 4.5 Upright Rows With Cords 60

No. 4.6 Punches With Cords 61

No. 4.10 Shoulder Flexion (with cords) 65

No. 5.12 Frontal Diagonal Pulls 98

Sidestroke on both sides of body

If you have chronic back pain, add the following exercise in addition to the global advanced program.

Backstroke or freestyle swimming. Breaststroke is appropriate at this stage.

If you have herniated discs, spondylolysis or spondylolisthesis, focus on the advanced level global program as it is presented. Continue with the sidestroke and deep water jogging. Avoid activities that involve repetitive rotation of the trunk or hyperextension. Concentrate on abdominal exercises to lend support to the back.

If you have unoperated scoliosis, add the following exercises in addition to the existing advanced global program.

No. 5.10 Cheerleading Squats 96

No 5.12 Frontal Diagonal Pulls (both sides) 98

No. 5.11 Upper Extremity PNF Diagonal (both sides) 97

Sidestroke, American crawl, or backstroke

If you have surgical scoliosis, follow the global programs throughout the beginner, intermediate, and advanced levels. Concentrate on strengthening the abdominals and back extensors. Avoid activities that involve bending the trunk forward or backward to extreme ranges and excessive or repetitive twisting of the trunk.

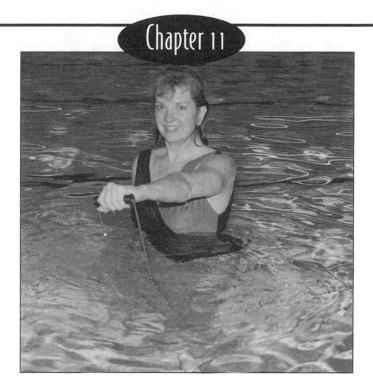

Chapter 11

Shoulder

This chapter covers shoulder pain resulting from soft tissue injury caused by trauma, poor posture, and muscle imbalances. All of these can lead to significant shoulder pain and loss of function if left unaddressed.

Shoulder dislocation results from a trauma to the body, such as occurs in a fall on an outstretched arm, or a direct blow to the area sustained in sports-related activities. Rotator cuff strains or impingement can result from muscle imbalances, or from faulty posture that leads to muscle imbalance. In other instances, rotator cuff strain may result from the decreased vascularity, or blood flow, to that area of the shoulder that occurs with advancing age. This decrease in blood flow gives rise to degenerative changes.

As in the other chapters, each shoulder condition is generally discussed. Then, a rehabilitation program of water exercises is presented in beginner, intermediate, and advanced level formats. Exercises are numbered so you can refer to Part II of this book to review each particular exercise and its precautions.

DISLOCATION OR SUBLUXATION

Shoulder dislocation or subluxation may be a one-time incident related to the application of excessive force or trauma to the shoulder complex. It might also be recurrent in nature, resulting in an unstable shoulder. One of the most vulnerable positions of the shoulder is abduction and external rotation. To simplify those terms, picture the posture of a baseball pitcher, quarterback, or javelin thrower prior to releasing the ball or javelin—that is abduction and external rotation. The arm and shoulder are cocked back near the ear with the upper arm level with the shoulder. Overuse injuries, or a fall with the arm in this position, can result in dislocation or subluxation. When subluxation occurs, pain and numbness may be felt, followed by weakness of the arm (*Modern Principles of Athletic Training*, Arnheim). The dislocation will need to be corrected by a physician or athletic trainer and then immobilized for several weeks in a sling. After that time, the physician must give clearance to begin rehabilitation.

The shoulder complex must be strengthened to ensure the stability of the joint. Water exercise allows rehabilitation with less pain because the limb is unweighted by the absence of gravity. Endurance and strength can be developed while the arm is supported through buoyancy.

ROTATOR CUFF STRAINS AND IMPINGEMENT

Rotator cuff strains and impingement may also occur from repetitive throwing motions or the loading of the shoulder complex in extreme external rotation and abduction. Again, that posture is common to baseball pitchers, quarterbacks, in the overhead tennis serve, and weightlifting with free weights. All these activities place the shoulder in a very vulnerable position. Swimmers commonly experience rotator cuff strains due to repetitive, overhead resistive actions. Freestyle and butterfly strokes result in overloading of the shoulder as well as muscle imbalances. Competitive swimmers may begin to experience rotator cuff strains around 18-20 years of age—depending on the level and duration of their competitive careers. Rotator cuff or impingement problems commonly occur in women 40-60 years of age without a specific related injury. This may be related to degenerative changes because of decreased bloodflow to the area.

The rotator cuff of the shoulder is a group of four muscles that attach in a cuff-like fashion around the head of the humerus, or upper arm, and are responsible for the internal (inward) and external (outward) rotation of the arm. Besides strengthening and resolving muscle imbalances around the shoulder complex, proper posture is equally important in avoiding rotator cuff strains or dysfunction.

With a rotator cuff strain, or any other dysfunctional shoulder condition, one must avoid the posture the body will subconsciously seek out—that of holding the arm flexed and cradled across the chest. Avoid this posture; it only compounds the dysfunction. At night, when pain or discomfort may be significant enough to wake you, do the following: Prop the arm up on 1-2 pillows when lying on your uninvolved side so that the involved arm is properly supported. This should help with the discomfort by preventing the involved shoulder from falling forward across the chest into the forbidden posture!

EXERCISE PROGRAMS

This program of water exercise, coupled with preventative measures such as those previously addressed, will result in a stronger, more stable shoulder. Persevere. Shoulder injuries require patience.* The following exercises are appropriate for the unstable shoulder and for rotator cuff strains.

Beginner Level

Perform one set of 15 repetitions (remaining 2-3 weeks at this level).

No. 3.1 Warm-Up Laps   26
No. 3.2 Sideways Walk   27

*Consult your physician and physical or occupational therapist about the resumption of overhead activities or the return to a sport that involves overhead motions.

No. 3.6 Biceps Curl   31

No. 3.9 Internal and External Shoulder Rotation   34

No. 3.8 Shoulder Press-Downs (above-the-waist water
with no paddles for resistance)   33

No. 3.10 Trunk Twists (above-the-water to ensure 90 degrees
or less of shoulder flexion)   35

No. 4.3 Wall Push-Ups (hands placed *below* shoulder level
to ensure 90 degrees or less of shoulder flexion)   58

No. 3.15 Bird (no barbells; in above-the-waist water to ensure
90 degrees or less of shoulder abduction)   40

No. 4.1 Alternate Press-Downs (in above-the-waist water to
ensure 90 degrees or less of shoulder flexion;
use no paddles)   56

No. 6.1 Deep Water Jogging (with upper extremity running
motion for range of motion exercise. Jog 5-10 min.)   108

Intermediate Level

Perform two sets of 12-15 repetitions and stay at this level 3-4 weeks.
Do not progress to Intermediate Level until you have no pain or difficulty with the Beginner Level exercises.

No. 3.1 Warm-Up Laps (Beginning)   26

No. 5.2 Carioca (Advanced)   88

No. 4.9 Biceps Curl (Intermediate)   64

No. 3.7 Chest Flys (above-the-waist to chest-high water
with hand paddles)   32

No. 3.8 Shoulder Press-Downs (above-the-waist to
chest-high water with hand paddles)   33

No. 3.13 Barbell Push-Pulls   38

No. 4.13 Internal and External Shoulder Rotation (Intermediate)
(use paddles only if you are pain-free with this
posture and motion)   68

No. 3.15 Bird (may use paddles or barbells, whichever
is more comfortable)   40

No. 3.14 Gorilla Press-Downs (above-the-waist to
          chest-high water, whichever is more comfortable)   39

No. 4.10 Shoulder Flexion   65

No. 4.11 Shoulder Abduction   66

No. 4.12 Shoulder Empty Can   67

No. 4.5 Upright Rows With Cords   60

No. 6.1 Deep Water Jogging (15 min.)   108

Advanced Level

Perform two sets of 15 repetitions. Proceed to this level if you can perform the Intermediate Level exercises with no pain or increase in symptoms and have close to full range of motion.

No. 5.1 Warm-Up Laps (Advanced)   87

No. 3.10 Trunk Twists (chest-high water)   35

No. 3.7 Chest Flys   32

No. 3.8 Shoulder Press-Downs (Beginning)   33

No. 3.13 Barbell Push-Pulls   38

No. 3.14 Gorilla Press-Downs   39

No. 3.15 Bird   40

No. 4.10 Shoulder Flexion   65

No. 4.11 Shoulder Abduction   66

No. 4.12 Shoulder Empty Can   67

No. 4.5 Upright Rows With Cords   60

No. 4.6 Punches With Cords   61

No. 5.11 Upper Extremity PNF Diagonal   97

No. 4.7 Side-Swipes With Paddle (both sides)   62

No. 3.5 Abdominal Press-Downs (Beginning)   30

No. 4.13 Internal and External Shoulder Rotation (Intermediate)
          (with paddles)   68

No. 6.1 Deep Water Jogging (15-20 min.)
          Sidestroke only   108

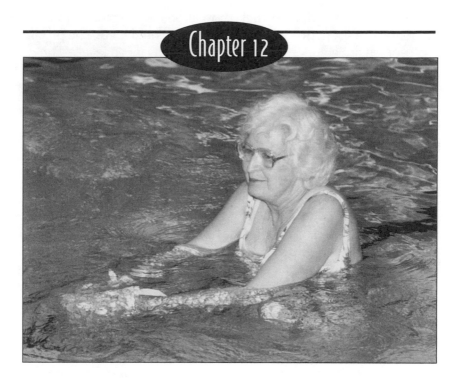

Elbow and Wrist

Chapter 12 includes a discussion of injuries common to the elbow and wrist. Epicondylitis, usually referred to as tennis elbow, may or may not be sports-related. It is a soft tissue disorder or response related to overuse. It may involve a racquet sport or result from a repetitive activity, such as hammering or chopping. It involves any repetitive activity where the wrist is hyperextended, or cocked back and up. It is usually a degenerative disorder resulting from a specific activity over a period of time. Common wrist injuries are also examined. Wrist fractures or dislocation primarily occur in older women and result from a fall on an outstretched arm and hand. This injury is seen more among women than men because of the prevalence of osteoporosis.

Following the overview of these conditions is a water exercise program to restore strength and flexibility to the injured area. The programs are presented in beginner, intermediate, and advanced levels. The exercises are numbered for easy reference to the exercise section in Part II of the book.

EPICONDYLITIS

Epicondylitis is an overuse syndrome known to many as tennis elbow or golfer's elbow and refers to the inflammation of the tendons that surround the lateral or outside bone beside the elbow.

Many racquet sports or sports that involve throwing lead to chronic overuse syndromes that develop over time from cumulative microtraumas. The injury occurs in sports that require repetitive turning of the forearm from a modified palm-up or open position to a rolling over and finishing movement or stroke where the palm is in a down-turned position. This syndrome is common in competitive athletic throwing or racquet sports, or in middle-aged athletes where degenerative changes from cumulative microtraumas over the years have developed. Management of epicondylitis first involves R-I-C-E: **R**est, **I**ce, **C**ompression, and **E**levation, or immobilization (if necessary). Many people have found a tennis or golfer's elbow strap helpful in managing their tendinitis. This is a small strap that applies pressure to the outside of the elbow. Also, if pain is persistent in the case of racquet sports, grip size and string tension should be investigated for appropriateness to hand size, strength, and level of competition.

Water exercise can help to resolve any muscle imbalances that may be contributing to the overload/overuse syndrome.

ELBOW AND WRIST FRACTURES

Elbow and wrist fractures are commonly caused by a fall on an outstretched hand with the elbow extended. There is immediate pain with accompanying swelling and sometimes bruising. The fracture of the wrist is known as Colles' fracture. In most cases, there is visible deformity, but occasionally it will be diagnosed as a badly sprained wrist. A Colles' fracture involves a period of immobilization through splinting or casting to allow for fracture healing. After the cast is removed, there will be pain and stiffness in the joint. This is to be expected. However, if there is an inordinate amount of pain, along with oversensitivity to light touch or temperature, consult a physician. Occasionally, a condition know as reflex sympathetic dystrophy (RSD) may be present and this will need to be addressed in a different way.

In the case of wrist and elbow injuries, you should concentrate on correcting muscle imbalances or inflexibilities to ensure proper and complete healing.

ELBOW DISLOCATIONS

Elbow dislocations require reduction by a physician as soon as possible to prevent secondary soft tissue and nerve compromise. Elbow fractures may not result in visible deformity, but will have the symptoms of swelling, possible bruising, and muscle spasms to prevent further movement of the joint. Consult your physician as soon as possible if you experience these symptoms.

EXERCISE PROGRAMS

Begin these exercises when cleared by your doctor, or physical or occupational therapist.

Beginner Level

Perform one set of 15 repetitions, continuing at this level for 2-4 weeks.

No. 3.1 Warm-Up Laps   26
No. 3.2 Sideways Walk   27
No. 3.7 Chest Flys (no paddles)   32
No. 3.8 Shoulder Press-Downs (no paddles)   33
No. 3.13 Barbell Push-Pulls   38
No. 3.14 Gorilla Press-Downs (no resistance)   39
No. 3.9 Internal and External Shoulder Rotation   34

No. 3.23 Wrist Curls (no resistance)   48

No. 6.1 Deep Water Jogging (5-15 min.)   108

Intermediate Level

Perform two sets of 15 repetitions and remain at this level for 2-4 weeks.
   Continue with all the Beginner Level exercises but add resistance (hand paddles).

No. 3.7 Chest Flys (hand paddles)   32

No. 3.8 Shoulder Press-Downs (Beginning; hand paddles)   33

No. 3.14 Gorilla Press-Downs (hand barbells)   39

No. 3.15 Bird (hand barbells)   40

No. 4.13 Internal and External Shoulder Rotation (Intermediate)   68

No. 3.23 Wrist Curls (hand paddles)   48

No. 4.4 Washboard   59

No. 4.3 Wall Push-Ups   58

No. 6.1 Deep Water Jogging (15 min.)   108

Advanced Level

Perform three sets of 15 repetitions.
   Continue with the Intermediate Level of exercises as presented. Add any swimming stroke to tolerance.

No. 4.7 Side-Swipes With Paddle   62

No. 3.5 Abdominal Press-Downs (Beginning)   30

Part IV

Programs for Total Fitness

I n the concluding section of *Water Exercise*, the use of water exercise for basic fitness, cross-training and special populations is addressed. Chapter 13 is for those individuals who want an exercise program that is effective, not too demanding, and easy to stay with over a period of time. The benefits to be derived from a basic water exercise program include overall toning, increased endurance, lowering of cholesterol, and, possibly, weight loss.

Chapter 14 is an advanced water exercise program for the individual who wants a challenging program with all the health benefits of the basic exercise program plus strengthening. Chapter 14's advanced water exercise program is appropriate for the serious, competitive athlete looking for an effective cross-training program. Water exercise is an excellent choice because it allows the body to recover from the wear and tear of competition safely while continuing to work in a resistive environment that can also challenge the cardiovascular system.

Chapter 15 covers the use of water exercise to meet the therapeutic needs of special populations that have one of the following conditions: rheumatoid arthritis, Parkinson's disease, osteoporosis, fibromyalgia, or multiple sclerosis. Their therapeutic goals are different from those of individuals addressing orthopedic problems, as presented in Part III,

Programs for Common Injuries. Over the years, my water therapy has provided good results for the conditions covered in chapter 15, Special Populations.

In the Basic Water Exercise Program covered in chapter 13, beginner and intermediate levels of water exercise are introduced. Chapter 14 deals with the advanced level exercises. Chapter 15 includes a beginner level of exercise with an abbreviated intermediate level of water exercises for special populations. All of these are numbered for easy reference in Part II of the book, with accompanying illustrations.

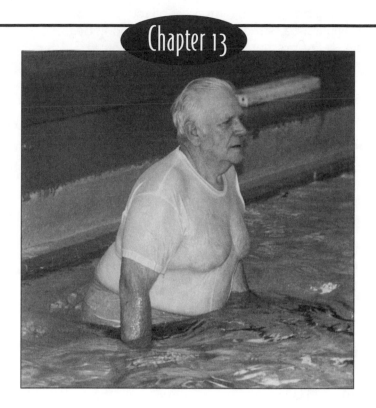

Chapter 13

Basic Water Exercise Program

Any complete exercise program will emphasize flexibility, endurance, strength, and coordination. A healthy, strong body will maintain a balance among these four components. Actually, these components provide the foundation upon which we build the body. If you are negligent in addressing any one of these areas, you could very well be setting yourself up for injury or performance problems in the future.

Fitness is multifaceted. You should not concentrate on only one dimension, like endurance or strength. It is a graded process: You start at the beginning and build on your flexibility and endurance, then progress to more demanding exercises without delays from minor or nagging injuries.

The following program encompasses all four components of fitness—flexibility, endurance, strength, and coordination. Beginner and intermediate levels are presented and should be followed 3-4 times a week. This program could be combined with a moderate walking, jogging, or biking program every other day for cross-training. Allow 1-3 rest days a week to let the body recover. Each session should last 45-90 minutes.

Beginner

Perform one set of 20 repetitions.

No. 3.1 Warm-Up Laps (5 min.)   26

No. 3.2 Sideways Walk (5 min.)   27

No. 3.3 High Kicks   28

No. 3.4 Hip In and Outs   29

No. 3.26 Heel Rock and Rolls   51

No. 3.5 Abdominal Press-Downs   30

No. 3.7 Chest Flys   32

No. 3.8 Shoulder Press-Downs   33

No. 3.10 Trunk Twists   35

No. 3.14 Gorilla Press-Downs   39

No. 3.15 Bird   40

No. 5.9 Squats   95

No. 4.27 Lunges (Intermediate)   82

No. 4.21 Lateral Trunk Flexion (Hula Dancer)   76

No. 3.21 Figure 8   46

No. 6.1 Water Jogging (15-20 min.)   108
        or Swimming (10-15 min.)

Intermediate

Perform two sets of 15 repetitions, 3-4 weeks later.

No. 5.1 Warm-Up Laps (Advanced)   87

No. 5.2 Carioca (Advanced)   88

No. 3.3 High Kicks (Beginning)   28

No. 3.4 Hip In and Outs (Beginning)   29

No. 3.5 Abdominal Press-Downs (Beginning)   30

No. 3.7 Chest Flys   32

No. 3.8 Shoulder Press-Downs (Beginning)   33

No. 4.1 Alternate Press-Downs   56

No. 4.7 Side-Swipes With Paddle   62

No. 4.5 Upright Rows With Cords   60

No. 4.6 Punches With Cords   61

No. 3.14 Gorilla Press-Downs   39

No. 3.15 Bird   40

No. 5.9 Squats With Ball   95

No. 4.27 Lunges (Intermediate)   82

No. 4.24 Bunny Hop   79

No. 4.29 Windmills   84

No. 6.1 Deep Water Jogging (20-30 min.)   108
         or Swimming (15-30 min.)

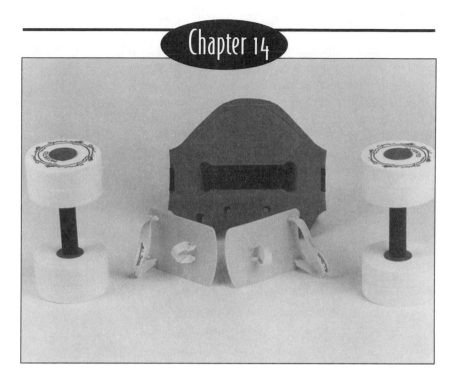

Chapter 14

Advanced Water Exercise Program

By the time you reach this level of the fitness program, you should either have progressed through the beginner and intermediate phases or be a competitive athlete in need of a good cross-training program. The advanced level water exercise program focuses on more demanding aerobic endurance work as well as strength training. You should do this workout every other day and should exercise consistently 5-6 days a week with 1-2 rest days interspersed in the program—possibly 1 midweek day and 1 weekend day.

In addition to a challenging cardiovascular workout, these advanced level water exercises emphasize strengthening by isolating specific muscle groups. This is one of the benefits of cross-training. This collection of exercises isolates every major muscle group, not just the one involved in your sport.

There is also a great deal of emphasis placed on trunk strength and control. If you have good trunk strength and control, you will be working from a strong and stable foundation. The stronger your foundation, the better the performance from those extensions off the trunk, the arms and legs. If you are not working from a strong foundation, it is just a matter of time before you develop some muscle imbalances or overuse injuries. The advanced water exercise program addresses overall flexibility, strengthening of all major muscle groups, trunk strength and stability, and cardiovascular endurance.

The following exercises are numbered for easy reference to Part II of the book on specific water exercises.

Perform three sets of 15 repetitions.

No. 5.1 Warm-Up Laps (Advanced)   87

No. 5.2 Carioca (Advanced)   88

No. 5.4 High Kicks (Advanced)   90

No. 5.5 Hip In and Outs (Advanced)   91

No. 3.5 Abdominal Press-Downs (Beginning)   30

No. 4.28 Sitting Abdominal and Hip Crunches   83

No. 5.9 Squats With Ball   95

No. 5.3 Lunges (Advanced)   89

No. 3.14 Gorilla Press-Downs   39

No. 3.15 Bird   40

No. 3.7 Chest Flys   32

No. 4.7 Side-Swipes With Paddle   62

No. 5.13 "X" Marks the Spot   99

No. 5.11 Upper Extremity PNF Diagonal   97

No. 4.9 Biceps Curl (Intermediate)   64

No. 4.14 Hip Extension With Cords (Pull-Backs)   69

No. 4.17 Hip Adduction With Cords (Pull-Ins)   72

No. 4.15 Hip Flexion With Cords (Pull-Forwards)   70

No. 4.16 Hip Abduction With Cords (Pull-Outs)   71

No. 5.16 Seated Surfer   102

No. 6.1 Deep Water Jogging (30 min.)   108
or Swimming nonstop (30-45 min.) freestyle, sidestroke, backstroke, or breaststroke, or a combination of all strokes.

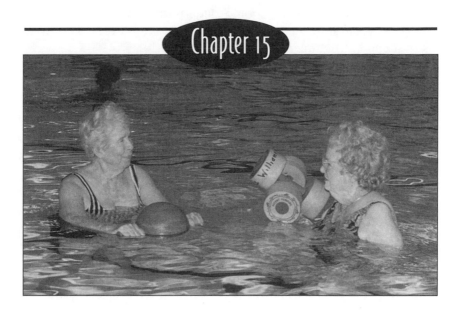

Chapter 15

Special Populations

Chapter 15 discusses individuals whose therapeutic needs are different from everything discussed up to this point in the book. This chapter will focus on rheumatoid arthritis, Parkinson's disease, osteoporosis, fibromyalgia, and multiple sclerosis. Rheumatoid arthritis, osteoporosis, and fibromyalgia are disorders of the arthritis family. Parkinson's disease and multiple sclerosis are systemic disorders that involve a dysfunction of the central nervous system.

The therapeutic goals are different for individuals who have any of these diseases. The degenerative processes are ongoing and the degree to which they affect individuals varies widely. That is why it is difficult to specifically address individual needs in this group of diseases. Therapeutically, however, the rehabilitative goals are universal. Through water exercise, one can slow the ongoing degenerative process, whether it involves the skeletal system or the central nervous system. Therapeutic goals that can be met include

- increased functional range of motion,
- increased overall endurance,
- increased functional strength,
- increased overall mobility,
- improved overall balance, and
- decreased dependence on others to assist in activities of daily living including dressing, grooming, bathing, and eating.

The water exercise program presented in this chapter is sufficient for meeting the above-mentioned goals for people with either rheumatoid arthritis, Parkinson's disease, osteoporosis, fibromyalgia, or multiple sclerosis. The program may be too easy for some people or too challenging for others. However, I feel it is a program that is reasonable for the majority of individuals dealing with any of the above-mentioned diseases. There is a modified intermediate level for those who need more from their water exercise program.

The symptoms and signs of all of these diseases vary widely. I strongly urge you to contact the national office as well as local chapters or support groups in these different disease groups. I have included toll-free national headquarters phone numbers or addresses for each specific disease included herein.

Any doctor you talk with about rheumatoid arthritis, Parkinson's disease, osteoporosis, fibromyalgia, or multiple sclerosis will tell you that some form of light exercise is imperative to slowing the disease process. In water, you have a safe and supportive environment, but also one that is resistive, so one's endurance and strength can be improved. I strongly urge you to participate, to your level of tolerance, 2-3 times a week, for 20-45 minutes in the water exercise program outlined in this chapter. It will make a difference both physically and psychologically.

Each exercise is numbered for your convenience and reference. Descriptions of the exercises appear in Part II of the book in chapters 3-6. If you have difficulty balancing, do these exercises with your back against the wall for added stability.

Also, with the water jogging, for those individuals who are able, jog without the belt in waist-high to chest-high water. The addition of a jogging or ski belt may make you too buoyant to keep your balance. Also, by jogging where you touch the pool floor, you get more weightbearing and input into the nervous system. This helps with your body awareness and knowing where you are in space, and this will help you with your balance. Jog very easy and rest as needed. Do not push yourself.

RHEUMATOID ARTHRITIS

Rheumatoid arthritis is a complex disease with a myriad of symptoms. It can affect young and old alike, but is more common between the ages of 20-50 years old. It has a higher incidence in women, with over 100 distinct disorders in the rheumatic family. According to John L. Calabro, M.D., in a *Clinical Symposia Report* on Rheumatoid Arthritis (Vol. 8, No. 2, 1986), the disease is systemic and can lead to proliferative and degenerative changes in the joints. Systemic manifestations are most common in children and can include high fevers, weight loss, rash, and unusual activities (due to joint pain). Joints commonly affected include the feet, ankles, wrists, elbows, shoulders, and knees.

Water therapy is excellent for those with rheumatoid arthritis because of the decreased stress and weightbearing on joints, as well as the support added through buoyancy. Range-of-motion exercises in all joints are an important phase of rehabilitation for these individuals. Because of the gravity-eliminated property of water, it is easier and less painful to exercise. Movement is important for maintaining strength and endurance, both of which are mandatory in staying one step ahead of this disease. Focus on joint range of motion and avoid exercises that increase or add resistance to the movement, as these can quickly aggravate symptoms.

For more information on rheumatoid arthritis, call the Arthritis Foundation at 1-800-283-7800, or your local chapter as listed in the business directory.

PARKINSON'S DISEASE (PARKINSONISM)

Parkinsonism was first discovered in 1817 by James Parkinson. In his essay (1817), he described Parkinsonism as a "chronic progressive disorder of the nervous system beginning in middle age." He described it further as a mild tremor and weakness of one hand that spreads later to other joints. Research studies over the years have helped Parkinsonism become less confusing and more treatable. Appropriate management through drug therapy is a huge part of the successful treatment of this disease.

Parkinsonism is a progressive disorder that goes through several stages. Balance impairment, slowness of body movements, and increasing rigidity affect the person with Parkinsonism. Through water therapy, this individual can move more easily in an environment that is gravity-free. The buoyancy of water offers additional support for balance. Range-of-motion exercises against the resistance of water keep the endurance up and overall mobility intact. Water exercise is comfortable and effective in the treatment of Parkinsonism.

For more information on Parkinsonism call the Parkinson Foundation at 1-800-457-6676, or call your local chapter as listed in the business directory.

OSTEOPOROSIS

Osteoporosis is a very common disorder of the elderly population and is the result of decreased bone mass. The skeletal system of the body can no longer withstand everyday stresses because of the compromised state of the bone mass due to mineral loss. The highest-risk group for osteoporosis is post-menopausal women. There is a high frequency of fractures at the hips, wrists, ribs, and thoracic (mid-back) and lumbar (low-back) vertebrae. There may also be a gradual loss of height and stooped posture, known as dowager's hump. Besides aging and hormonal deficiencies, poor diet, alcoholism, heavy cigarette smoking, and a sedentary lifestyle also contribute to osteoporosis.

Because the skeletal system's ability to withstand normal mechanical stresses is compromised, water exercise is a safe and effective means of overall strengthening. Decreased compressive forces, supportive buoyancy, a gravity-eliminated environment, and the resistive property of water make the pool an excellent overall resource for building strength and trunk stabilization safely. Calcium supplements, hormonal drugs, daily walking, or mild exercise are essential to maintaining existing bone mass. For more information on osteoporosis, contact the National Osteoporosis Foundation, Box 96173, Washington, DC, 20077-7456.

FIBROMYALGIA

Fibromyalgia is a fairly recent entity and has remained controversial since its recognition by the medical community. Dr. Janet Travell and Dr. David Simons launched the recognition and treatment of fibromyalgia with their book *Myofascial Pain and Dysfunction* in 1983. They describe myalgia as "1) diffusely aching muscles due to systemic disease, such as a virus infection and 2) the spot tenderness of a muscle(s) as in trigger points." Their clinical studies found people between the ages of 31 and 50 years to be most widely affected. Fibromyalgia has also been described as muscular rheumatism, and is in fact listed under the rheumatic family. Consistent symptoms include diffuse muscular pain present longer than 3 to 4 months, localized tenderness, and disturbed sleep with morning fatigue and stiffness (J. Travell, M.D., and D. Simons, M.D., 1983). Just about everyone has had these symptoms at one time or another and that is why fibromyalgia remains controversial. However, with fibromyalgia, these symptoms are ongoing as opposed to temporary in nature.

Because these individuals are prone to tendinitis, bursitis, and diffuse muscular pain in association with exercise, the water is a safer, more comfortable environment in which to exercise. Again, the many properties of water make it ideal for those populations that have special needs and concerns. The goals of strengthening, increased range of motion, correction of postural dysfunction, and gains in endurance are achievable with water exercises.

For more information on fibromyalgia, contact the Arthritis Foundation at 1-800-283-7800, or your local chapter or support groups as listed in the business directory.

MULTIPLE SCLEROSIS

Multiple sclerosis is a disorder of the central nervous system in which the lining of the nerve is disturbed or destroyed. As this lining degenerates over a period of time, it is replaced by scar tissue. This process impairs the efficiency of the nerve and leads to the characteristic rapid fatigue found with multiple sclerosis. There are no classic neurologic signs with multiple sclerosis other than a history of previous mild attacks, remission, then exacerbation of symptoms. There are gross motor disturbances, which vary in intensity with each individual. Significant problems with balance and walking are characteristic of this disease. These can range from mild to debilitating. Heat is fatiguing to individuals with multiple sclerosis and can even push them to the point of exhaustion. Jacuzzis, hot tubs, and hot baths should be avoided. According to René Calliet, M.D., in "Exercise in Multiple Sclerosis" (*Therapeutic Exercise*, fourth edition, 1984), there are four clinical classifications of multiple sclerosis that are recognized, and these vary widely. Also, exercise plays a vital role in the treatment of multiple sclerosis, but the exercise program must fit the individual in accordance with his or her neurological deficit. Increased muscle tone (spasticity) affects gross motor performance and this varies according to the degree of impairment in the central nervous system.

Water exercise offers a supportive, buoyant environment to these individuals. Warm water (84-88 degrees) helps inhibit spasticity and allows for easier movement. Working in chest-high water makes the individual less weightbearing because of buoyancy. This reduces spasticity in the legs and allows greater ease in walking. Coordination is improved through the repetition of the water exercises. Inactivity will lead to a rapid loss of coordination (R. Calliet, M.D., *Therapeutic Exercise*, fourth edition, 1984).

While there is no reversing this degenerative process, exercise in water enables the individual to be more independent and functional. One can improve in overall strength, endurance, and coordination because of the therapeutic properties of water.

For more information on multiple sclerosis, call the Multiple Sclerosis Foundation at 1-800-441-7055, or check the business pages for your local chapter.

Beginner Level

Perform one set of 10-15 repetitions.

No. 3.1 Warm-Up Laps   26
No. 3.2 Sideways Walk   27
No. 3.3 High Kicks   28

No. 3.20 Hip Abduction Facing Wall   45

No. 3.26 Heel Rock and Rolls   51

No. 3.10 Trunk Twists   35

No. 3.12 Knee to Chest   37

No. 3.7 Chest Flys   32

No. 3.8 Shoulder Press-Downs   33

No. 3.6 Biceps Curl   31

No. 3.23 Wrist Curls   48

Intermediate Level

Perform one set of 20 repetitions.

Continue with all exercises in the Beginner Level and add these exercises.

No. 4.4 Washboard   59

No. 3.9 Internal and External Shoulder Rotation (Beginning)   34

No. 4.3 Wall Push-Ups   58

No. 3.11 Marching in Place   36

No. 6.1 Deep Water Jogging (up to 15 min.—rest as needed)   108

Index

About the Author

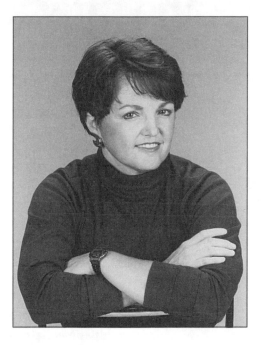

Martha D. White specializes in developing water therapy programs for orthopedic, rheumatic, and musculoskeletal conditions and diseases. She served as the occupational therapist in Baylor College of Medicine's outpatient chronic pain management program from 1986 to 1988. Since 1990 she has been developer and director of the aquatic therapy program for the outpatient sports medicine clinic at the Texas Medical Center in Houston. Most recently, Martha's work has focused on diversifying her water therapy programs to meet the needs of special populations.

Martha is a licensed occupational and massage therapist as well as a member of the Aquatic Exercise Association and the National Strength and Conditioning Association. For leisure, Martha enjoys water sports, jogging, reading, and spectator sports in her hometown of Houston, Texas.

More books for safe and effective exercise

Water Fitness After 40

Ruth Sova

Foreword by Julie See

1995 • Paper • Approx 200 pp • Item PSOV0604
ISBN 0-87322-604-6 • $15.95 ($22.50 Canadian)

Slow the aging process and stay fit for years to come. This book provides everything you need to create a personalized, pain-free water fitness program.

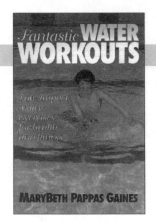

Fantastic Water Workouts

MaryBeth Pappas Gaines

1993 • Paper • 184 pp • Item PGAI0458
ISBN 0-87322-458-2
$14.95 ($20.95 Canadian)

Contains 90 water exercises that are fun, effective, and easy on your body. All of the exercises make creative use of water's natural buoyancy and resistance to give you maximum results with a minimum risk of injury.

Price subject to change.

To place an order: U.S. customers call **TOLL-FREE 1 800 747-4457**; customers outside of U.S. use the appropriate telephone number/address shown in the front of this book.

Human Kinetics

2335

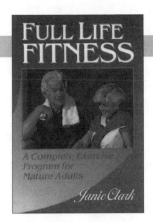

Full Life Fitness

*A Complete Exercise Program
for Mature Adults*

Janie Clark

**1992 • Paper • 192 pp • Item PCLA0391
ISBN 0-87322-391-8 • $13.95 ($17.50 Canadian)**

Enjoy the benefits of physical exercise while avoiding fatigue and overexertion. Featuring only low-stress and no-stress exercises, this book helps mature adults at all fitness levels find the fitness program that's right for them.

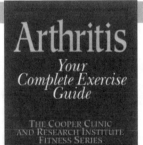

Arthritis

Your Complete Exercise Guide

[The Cooper Clinic and Research Institute Fitness Series]

Neil F. Gordon, MD, PhD, MPH

Foreword by Kenneth H. Cooper, MD, MPH

**1993 • Paper • 152 pp • Item PGOR0392
ISBN 0-87322-392-6 • $11.95 ($15.95 Canadian)**

Exercise your way to a healthier lifestyle! This book provides a safe and sensible exercise program that will help reduce the adverse effects of arthritis and improve fitness.

Other titles in The Cooper Clinic and Research Institute Fitness Series

*Breathing Disorders: Your Complete Exercise Guide
Chronic Fatigue: Your Complete Exercise Guide
Diabetes: Your Complete Exercise Guide
Stroke: Your Complete Exercise Guide*